I0041163

AVOIDING Attendants from HELL

A Practical Guide

To

Finding, Hiring & Keeping

Personal Care Attendants

2nd Edition

June Price

Science & Humanities Press
PO Box 7151
Chesterfield, MO 63006-7151
(636) 394-4950

Cover and internal drawings by Barry Whitesell.

ISBN 1-888725-60-5 Paperback

Library of Congress Cataloging-in-Publication Data
Price, June, 1947- Avoiding attendants from hell : a practical guide to finding, hiring & keeping personal care attendants / June Price.-- 2nd ed.
    p. cm.
    ISBN 1-888725-60-5 (Library/School Edition : alk. paper)
    -- ISBN 1-888725-72-9 (accessible plastic comb binding : alk. paper)
    1. Physically handicapped--Home care. 2. Home health aides--Selection
    and appointment. I. Title.
    HV3011 .P75 2001
    362.1'4--dc21
                                        2001006346

Science & Humanities Press
PO Box 7151
Chesterfield, MO 63006-7151
(636) 394-4950
sciencehumanitiespress.com

Dedication

This book is dedicated to all of my fellow comrades-in-arms in the war of independence — a war we fight daily. May you find the strength to fight another day, as I have, with the help and support of those who share in our struggles to maintain this freedom.

To the "saving graces" — the caring women who have helped me maintain my independence for almost two decades. You have given me far more than a bath and change of clothes. Some of you, especially dear, have provided lifelong memories of good times, compassionate care and special friendships that will forever warm my heart and get me through difficult days.

And to my parents who continue to provide the nuts and bolts of my independence—both literally and figuratively. Their love, help and support are unparalleled.

Table of Contents

Introduction

For many, the dream of living independently turns into a nightmare when working relationships with Personal Care Attendants (PCAS) do not work out as hoped. Good workers are, indeed, hard to find — even harder to keep.

Most people believe that if they were rich and famous — like Christopher Reeve — they would have no problem finding quality Personal Care Attendants. But, in all likelihood, Reeve struggles with the same issues as the rest of us do who are physically dependent on others for their daily care.

- **Finding** people to provide quality personal care requires the nose of a Bloodhound.
- **Hiring** them requires the investigative skills of Sherlock Holmes.
- **Keeping** them requires little less than an act of God.

The following guidelines can help you avoid ending up with an "attendant from Hell." With good planning and a little luck you can live happily ever after in the Land of Independent Living!

Who Should Move Out

The prospect of moving into one's own apartment is both exciting and terrifying. When the opportunity was first presented to me, I was told of two apartment vacancies. I would take one of the units and my friend, Jim, would take the other.

We spent weeks discussing how we would manage because we had similar needs and limitations. We were anxious to move though knew problems surely lay ahead.

I called Jim the night before we were to sign the rental lease to confirm our meeting. With great hesitation, he told me he had changed his mind and would, instead, move to an isolated town with his retiring parents. Jim was, admittedly, too afraid to move out on his own.

In the end, this was the right decision for Jim. And my decision to go ahead with the move turned out to be the right one for me.

◆•◈•◆

This is not a lifestyle for the faint-of-heart and may not be right for you. Deciding against moving into your own apartment can be wise if you are not up to its daily challenges. For some, other options may be better: living with family, residing in a group home, or even finding a nursing home which provides the care and socialization that meets your needs. Although these might not at first appear to be the most glamorous alternatives, independent living is by no means a walk on the beach.

Make sure this challenging lifestyle is right for you before making a leap you may one day regret.

Chapter 1

Getting Started

Some disabled individuals believe a Personal Care Assistant (PCA) will come to them like Mary Poppins did — floating down from the sky with a big smile and good heart — just when they need her the most. Unfortunately, that ain't gonna happen. Instead, finding a PCA requires a lot of time, skill and hard work.

Begin by calling your local Center for Independent Living (CIL) for assistance, information and support. Keep in mind you are not their only consumer. You may get faster results if you assist with the phone calling and other work.

Examine your needs by asking yourself some specific questions before proceeding:

◆ What are my care needs? Make a complete list.

◆ When do I need help? Morning and night but not days? Days but not nights? Just overnight? 24-hours a day?

◆ How many people will it take to fulfill my care needs per day/week?

- What kind of help am I looking for? Strictly personal care? Companionship? Housekeeping? A combination?
- How much funding is available to pay for help, or how much can I personally afford to pay?
- Can I offer additional benefits? Free room, shared rent, board?
- Will I hire only a man or only a woman, or is either gender acceptable?
- Is race or ethnicity a consideration?
- Are there any personal qualities I need or prefer in a PCA? Strength, gentleness, ambitiousness, patience, an independent thinker, easily directed?
- Can my PCA have a disability? Hearing loss, under/overweight, gait impairment, cognitive disability, artificial limb?
- Can I hire a foreign-speaking individual?
- Will I hire a minor? Some funding sources prohibit this.
- Will I hire a smoker?
- Must the PCA have her own car? Drive my vehicle? Drive me in theirs?

Once your PCA profile is developed, you will be able to seek out the best resources for finding help. For example, it may be a waste of time to advertise at a college if you need 24-hour care. However, this may be the ideal place to find occasional or part-time help.

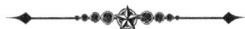

◆ —••◈••— ◆

Develop a flyer specifying job requirements. [See Appendix A] Also, **place want ads** [See Appendix B]. Consider these sources for posting flyers or ads:

- city and community newspapers
- college newspapers and bulletin boards
- churches (bulletins and verbal announce-ments)
- Division of Vocational Rehabilitation
- community/recreation centers
- youth centers
- senior centers (seniors are age 55 and up!)
- fitness centers
- grocery store bulletin boards

Word of mouth is often your best advertising tool. People who know you can sell the job to people they know. Send flyers to anyone who can spread the word to others, especially friends or acquaintances in the health field (nurses, therapists, etc.). I even send flyers to my veterinarian and to the health store I frequent! People who have contact with a lot of people are our best resource.

Tell your disabled friends you are seeking a PCA. They may know of a qualified worker looking for employment.

Ask to make a short announcement to a particular group (i.e. church, school, recreation center). People are more apt to show interest once they meet you.

You must have a clear idea of the type of worker you are seeking and the duties you need them to perform before you can move on to the next step.

Chapter 2

Electronic Advertising

Computers and the Internet have had a dramatic impact on the lives of those of us with disabilities. Take correspondence, as one example. No longer do we need help opening, folding, addressing, and sending our mail. Now we can e-mail, fax and even "chat" *--independently and privately--*with little more than a few clicks on a keyboard.

Likewise, computers and the Internet can make advertising for a PCA equally as fast, independent, and private!

Traditionally, this tedious task involved extensive time, personnel, and expense. Placing a newspaper ad could run $100 per week. Making flyers involved first designing them, then having someone make copies, and finally finding other people to post them. Two weeks could easily pass before the first responses came in.

As for *privacy*, there was none. Between the people involved in making and posting the flyers, to the flyers in your home and those posted around town, to phone call responses... everyone knew you were looking for a PCA! Good luck if you needed to find a new worker without your current one knowing!

Electronic advertising, however, changes all this. These ads come in many forms, from "spam" (those unsolicited e-mails selling us everything from golf balls to pornography) to the banners and pop-up ads which clutter our screen when we're on the 'Net. They're the 21st Century "billboard," and they can be our new best friend when it comes to finding a PCA! I've used this method exclusively for the past year with 100% success--and I haven't spent a dime on ads, made a single flyer, or required the assistance of even one person in making copies or posting ads.

The simplest form of electronic advertising is by e-mailing. I don't mean annoying "spam." Here's how it works:

Develop a clear and concise job description to put in e-mail form. Avoid fancy fonts, colors, and borders. This is a want ad, not a Picasso! You want it read by the greatest number of people with the least amount of distractions.

Highlight the job description in the Subject line:

Subject: PART-TIME CAREGIVER SOUGHT

Follow with a summation of your needs:

Spinal cord injured, professional woman seeks caregiver to assist with overnight personal care two weekend per month.

List details. Double-space between each clear, easy-to-read item. Include all pertinent information:

- Job description

- Pay

- Hours

- Days

- Experience required

- Additional requirements (e.g. "Must be strong enough to fully lift and transfer 120 lb. person." "Must be able to drive me in my van.")

- Location (general area of city)

- Perks (e.g. "Clean, quiet, safe, security-locked apartment building in nice neighborhood. Lot parking. On bus line. Sleep in private room. Ideal study setting for students. Cable TV.")

- Additional information (i.e. Is smoking allowed? Do you have pets?)

- Start date

- Contact information (include e-mail and/or phone).

Write an introductory e-mail to your friends and acquaintances. (This will be e-mailed in addition to the job notice.) Tell them about your situation

and what you'd like from them:
Hi, everyone!

> As many of you know, my weekend respite aide, Kim, will be leaving me soon to get married. As of now, I've still not found her replacement.

> I've developed a job description for this position and am sending it to you in a second e-mail. I'm hoping you can help me by forwarding it to anyone and everyone you know. Please ask that they forward it, as well. Don't limit it to those who may be right for the job, just send it to everyone, as we never know who they might know who might be just right for this position!

> Thank you!

> Sarah

Targeting a specific population is another way of making your e-mail job notices even more effective! How would you like to have your job notice appear in the e-mailbox of every nursing or physical therapy student at a particular university, as example? It's not as hard as you'd think!

College and university staff have the capability of forwarding an e-mail to any or all students. Your job notice could be sent to all of the students at the college or just those within a specific department. Finding a faculty member or staff person willing to accommodate your request to electronically post an ad may not be easy, but it's definitely not impossible. Here's how to pursue it:

Most schools list departments and faculty on their Web site, often with e-mail addresses. Contact instructors who specialize in disability issues. Since many instructors look for guest speakers, you might offer to speak in their class in exchange for help in posting your ad.

As a side note when determining which students to target as potential PCAs, don't limit yourself to nursing, as example. Personally, I've had the least luck with nursing students, even though there is a nursing school one block away from me! Widen your search to include students in vocational rehabilitation, exercise science, and therapeutic recreation, as well as all the allied health specialties.

E-mailing is the fastest way to get the word out. I've written an ad in the morning, had it posted by noon, and gotten responses before dinner!

E-mail advertising can provide e-mail responses! Students don't have to feel uncomfortable making that first phone call inquiry. They can e-mail questions, and you can e-mail clear, detailed responses. You could even add a photo or link to your Web site (but only if you feel this would be a strong selling point).

Electronic advertising is not exclusive to college campuses, however. Myriad sites offer boundless opportunities for placing ads online. Here are some examples:

   ♦ **Some Web sites list consumers seeking workers and PCAs looking for work, often**

by city and/or state. To locate these sites, use a search engine to find "disability resources," "independent living," or even "caregiver," but not "PCA," as this will lead you to everything but Personal Care Attendants! All of the sites I've seen are free for those who search their lists or register their need for a caregiver.

♦ **Many colleges, universities, trade schools, community newspapers and bulletin boards** now offer electronic listings of job opportunity. Search your city and the words "classifieds" or "want ads." Or call local newspapers and ask if they have online listings.

♦ **Housing listings can also be an excellent resource!** Place your ad for a live-in position under "Rooms to Rent." Word your ad accordingly: "FREE ROOM and salary in exchange for part-time care of disabled person..."

Carefully screen these applicants to separate those who might be desperate for housing. However, don't be surprised if you find that perfect match for your needs--*and theirs!*

Let's enthusiastically embrace electronic advertising, as we now have an independent, fast, and private means of searching for PCAs!

Chapter 3

Preliminary Screening for a Live-In

We are often tempted to hire the first respondent who comes along — especially when we're desperate — but doing so will only result in getting stuck with that dreaded "attendant from Hell"!

Most applicants seek a live-in position for the housing and income, not because they love the work. An 18-year-old male once pleaded for me to hire him even though he didn't have any experience. After a lot of questioning, I learned that his mother had kicked him out of the house forcing him to live in his car in the middle of winter! Anything was better than this in his mind!

Be wary of an applicant's "extra baggage." Most adults, by age 30, have a home or apartment, a spouse, children, pets, furniture, and/or job goals. A live-in position might typically offer a 9' x 10' bedroom which allows the live-in to bring little more than a few boxes of possessions. My first county case worker told me, "I never met a live-in attendant who didn't bring a lot of extra baggage... and I don't mean Samsonite." There may be reasons many of these folks don't have the normal trappings of home, family and so on. They may end up being exceptional caregivers, but it would be prudent for you to find out what those reasons are.

Don't be too friendly on the phone. We are quick to set up an interview, thinking we're halfway home if we get the applicant in the door. However, without adequate preliminary screening, what we may get for our efforts is disappointment, wasted time and possibly worse. We're so careful not to give out our address and phone number to total strangers, yet we invite these same strangers to sit on our couch and tour our apartment while we tell them how vulnerable we are!

Screening means identifying good prospects while eliminating the rest. After the caller says, "I'm calling about the job you had advertised," don't babble on about yourself, the job, where you live, and so on. Instead say, "Yes, what did you need to know?" Their response will tell you what their primary interest is. If their first question is, "How much does this job pay?" or, "How much time off do I get?" it may be that you are not their number one interest.

Ask open-ended questions like, "Tell me about yourself." Although this may leave some folks fumbling for words, their response is often revealing.

Explain your needs. Ask tough questions while interspersing job information. For example I say, "I weigh only 95 lbs. but must be lifted cradle style, under my legs and around my back — like a man would carry his bride over a threshold. Is this something you feel you can do?" If they say, "Of course I

16

can lift you! I've lifted 250 lb. men!" it is clear they didn't listen or understand you. I then say, "You did a pivot transfer. I can't stand at all..." Keep following

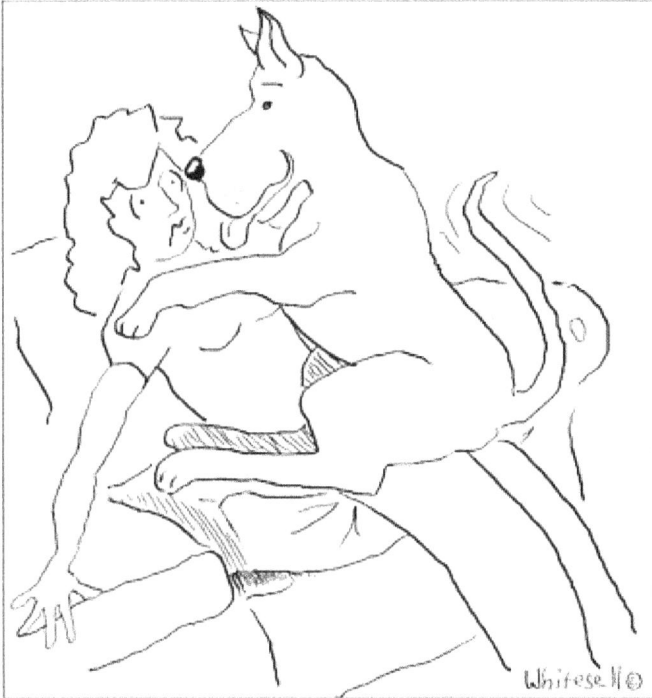

Ask how the applicant feels about living with pets...

up on the question until you are convinced they understand your needs and can meet them.

Must the person live in? Some people apply for a live-in position but don't think this must be their actual residence. Instead, they look at it as a part-time or third shift job. What are your requirements? Make sure they understand. Does the applicant expect someone to move in with them like their partner or child?

Clarify job duties, pay and time-off. Explain your personal care, cooking, housekeeping, shopping and other needs. State the pay rate and amount of time off.

Ask how the applicant feels about living with pets if you have any. "I don't mind as long as they leave me alone," is usually an indication the person doesn't like pets. Applicants have told me they "love" cats yet ignore mine in an interview! Living with someone who doesn't like pets can be traumatizing for both you and the pet.

Ask what the applicants like to do in their free time. One of my red flags is when someone says, "I just like to go out a lot during the day." Does that mean they are a nature lover, a Jehovah's Witness... or a drug dealer?

The goal is to screen out inappropriate respondents on the phone. This may sound harsh when we are desperate for help, but it is far worse to allow inappropriate applicants into our homes or hire them today only to fire them tomorrow.

The last step in preliminary screening is to "work" your key prospects. Don't make an interview appointment on the first call. Instead, call them back, even as early as the next day, to set up a date. This gives the applicant a chance to digest what was discussed while giving you the opportunity to eliminate spontaneous callers. When you call the second time, ask if the applicant is still interested. If so, set up a mutually agreed upon time and day for an interview. Tell the applicant to call if they change their mind about coming. Failure to call or show indicates irresponsible — the last thing we need.

Getting countless responses to your ad means nothing. What matters is the one to three good prospects. Screen out the rest and you won't be sorry.

Chapter 4

Initial In-Person Interview

Your apartment has been cleaned and you are well-groomed. You   are hopeful but nervous as the hour nears for your interview with a prospective **live-in attendant.**

The appointment time comes and goes, but no one shows. You confirmed the time just last night! Where are they? After 30 minutes, you decide to call.

"Hello. Is Rhonda there?" I asked the man who answered. "Just a minute," he gruffly says. "Rhonda? Hey, Rhonda — phone!" you hear in the background. "Who is it?" he bursts in. "June Price," I answer. "June Price," he shouts to another. There is a moment of silence before he returns, "She's not here." (Yes, this really happened!)

What causes this last minute change of heart? Frankly, it is indicative of the type of job we offer — to them, a small step above working at Burger King. This is frightening from our perspective, as this "job" is critical to our independence! But, although we'd like to think the person to whom we entrust our life will forever be loyal to us, the reality is that most won't. I'm reminded of a cat poem that read, "If I knew the lady next door would feed me better,

I'd be out of here in a minute. If you want loyalty, get a dog." Remember, to most applicants, this is just a job.

Lesson #1: Many job applicants will fail to show up for the interview. It's nothing against you; it's just that Burger King called last night offering them higher pay with fewer hours. Be grateful they didn't accept your job then change their mind.

Concentrate on the prospects who do show up! Note the following:

- ♦ **How timely was the applicant?** Being late is not good, but neither is being too early. It's important our worker has a watch and knows how to use it.

- ♦ **How well-groomed was the applicant?** If someone arrives dirty and unkempt for a job interview, do you really think they will keep you neat and clean? Think again.

- • **How appropriately-dressed was the applicant?**

  Thelma interviewed with me while remaining bundled in a coat, gloves, hat and scarf, refusing to remove any of these even after several requests. I don't know what her problem was, but I wasn't interested in pursuing a living and working relationship with someone this "closed."

  Silvia, a buxom blond, showed up in a sheer blouse, partially unbuttoned. Coupled with her long, wild hair and excessive make-up, I was taken aback. I might have excused her appearance had she not said, "I've got a lot of job interviews set up today!" I decided I was not interested in someone whose perception of appropriateness was so misguided!

♦ **How easily did the applicant find your residence?** Did they have difficulty finding your apartment? What skills did they employ to get there? Did they get lost finding your apartment building? Or even your door? We need people who can take direction and who have good problem solving skills!

♦ **How did the applicant approach you, if at all?** Did they eagerly offer to shake your hand? If so, give that person a gold star! On the other hand, if they hardly gave you eye contact, how can you expect them to be comfortable with your intimate care? Even initially, the applicant should feel comfortable in your presence. Be aware of body language. If they sit with arms or legs crossed, they may be concealing information. Someone who leans toward you and looks you straight in the eye is generally more open and honest.

♦ **How does the applicant respond to your home or apartment?** Comments about their surroundings often indicates a broader focus and awareness which is a desirable quality to have in a worker.

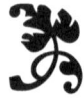

Chapter 5

The Job Application

Have the applicant complete a job application including her full name, permanent mailing address, date of birth, social security   number,   driver's license, last three jobs (include dates worked, company name, address, phone, supervisor, reason for leaving), personal references (non-friend or relative), and why they want the job. [See Appendix C]

I'm amazed how many disabled employers don't even know the spelling of their worker's last name. Keep this information in a permanent file. You will need it.

♦ **Make sure you have a permanent address**, not just a school or current address. A post office box will do. You will need this at tax time to forward mail or to send their last check after they leave.

♦ **Date of birth, social security number and driver's license are imperative** for verifying identity and checking for a criminal record.

♦ **Run a criminal check on the applicant**. Contact the Criminal Records Division of the county in which you live to get Felony Records Information. Someone must go in person for the records, but it need not be you. In some cases, a fee is involved.

- **Check driving records** through the Department of Motor Vehicles. In some cases, the applicant needs to sign a release for information and there may be a fee, but this is critical information to have. Even if your PCA will never drive your vehicle, the report can say a great deal about character and lifestyle when considering such infractions as a DUI/DWI, reckless use of a vehicle or revoked license.

- **Carefully scrutinize job references.** Some red flags include applicants who "can't remember" the name of a supervisor or other critical information as well as applications that reflect large gaps between jobs or short-term stays. Some people display a job record showing they worked three weeks here and two months there but say they plan to stay with you "for as many years as you need me!" I think not!

- **Beware of an applicant who can't provide personal references.** Some have told me they don't know anyone. I suggest a teacher, pastor or neighbor. If this still does not prompt a name, consider it another red flag. Reputable people have reputable references.

- **Why does the applicant want this job?** Is this the same reason they gave you on the phone? What is their main focus: housing, money, experience? Are there hidden reasons? Find out!

A job application is a valuable tool but it is useless if not scrutinized. Go over dates and other information then call their references.

Be advised that businesses are under no legal obligation to provide any information regarding former employees but may verify work dates.

You may get better results by calling personal references. I always let these contacts know that I'm physically disabled and totally vulnerable to those whom I hire. I ask them to please give me their honest opinion about the applicant, assuring them I will never divulge the source of information they provide.

With that, I've received some absolutely frightening information from people considered to be good friends of the applicant as well as some former employers. I've been told of drug problems, poor job records, and theft. In one instance, the applicant provided a reference who turned out to be a disabled woman I know. The applicant, it turned out, had worked for the woman only once but she knew of others for whom she had worked. She called those people for me and reported all were highly dissatisfied with the worker.

Checking references pays off every time!

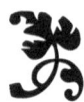

Chapter 6

The Interview — In Depth

You've gotten your first impressions of the live-in applicant, but for all you know, they may be an ax murderer. For all they know, you may be hell on wheels! How do you get beyond the surface to learn more about this prospective worker?

- ◆ **Ease the tension**. Compliment them for showing up. "I really appreciate you coming on such a snowy day!" or, "It must have taken forever to get here by bus. Thanks so much for coming!" Putting them at ease will create a more relaxed interviewing atmosphere. Offer water or a soft drink if you wish, but never offer an alcoholic beverage, nor should you be drinking one.

- ◆ **Ask the applicant to tell you about themselves.** It's everyone's favorite topic! Ask what they are currently doing and what led them to this job. Have them elaborate on their present schooling or employment. Listen for contradictions to what you were previously told. Hear potential problems. One applicant said she could move in immediately since she wasn't going to give her current disabled employer notice as she "didn't want that job anymore." That was all I needed to hear.

- ♦ **Redefine your needs.** You might say, "I explained what this job entails when we spoke by phone. Tell me what you understand the job to be." This will let you know what they've heard and understood. Describe a typical day — what tasks are expected of them and which are not.

- ♦ **It is imperative your job description be well-defined!** If you are not clear on what you need from a PCA, your needs will not be met, and the employee may become frustrated and quit. Those who have a newly-acquired or progressive disability often fail to recognize increasing needs.

One quad tells applicants he simply needs to be "thrown in his chair in the morning" (an agency home health aide does his personal care), and "thrown in bed at night." The reality is that he needs repositioning during the night, three meals a day, laundry, cleaning, shopping, banking, computer set-up, his van driven, and so on. Furthermore, when he has skin break-downs, he spends weeks or months in bed, requiring 24-hour care. When hospitalized (often for months at a time), his live-in does not get paid. He does not tell the applicant any of this ahead of time then wonders why those he hires quit so abruptly. He does not get "lousy aides", he simply gives lousy interviews.

♦ **Reiterate your living requirements.** Can anyone else move in with them? Can they bring a pet? What is included — rent, utilities, food, phone, cable? Do you provide the furniture in their room, or do they? Can they bring a waterbed? Can they put their table or chair in your living room? How much of the total apartment space can they use? Specify how many of your kitchen appliances and items they can use (i.e. microwave, toaster, dishes, pans, flatware, glasses).

♦ **How much free time does the applicant get?** Does every other weekend mean they are off Friday night until Monday morning? Saturday morning until Sunday night? Can they sleep in their room on days off, or are they expected to be off the premises completely? Are days off negotiable or set? What if they want more or less time off? How late can they stay out at night? Will the number of days off affect their pay?

♦ **How much freedom will the applicant have within your apartment?** Can they have guests over for dinner or have parties in the living room or must they stay in their bedroom? Are overnight guests permitted? If so,

31

how many and how often? Need they seek your permission before having guests?

♦ **Repeat your house rules regarding smoking, alcohol and drug use.** Reinforce your house rules.

♦ **Are there any potentially uncomfortable tasks you expect of them** such as giving you body massages, positioning you in bed with a sexual partner, or holding a marijuana cigarette for you to smoke? Be up front with your needs and requests, realizing not all PCAS are comfortable performing some tasks.

♦ **Ask if the applicant is in a relationship.** If so, how does their partner feel about their applying for this job? What effect might this job have on their relationship? Is it okay if their partner spends time at your apartment? If so, how often is okay with you—once a week? all weekend? most of the time? And what about you? Let them know if you are in a relationship. Would it bother them if you had someone stay overnight with you?

♦ **Are there any issues which may be sensitive with either of you?** Sexual preference, racial bias, religious practices can sometimes be major barriers when living under the same roof. Be honest now—or sorry later.

♦ **Don't assume anything!** The above is just a hint of the details which must be discussed in an interview to determine lifestyle compatibility and serious house rules. Make a list of everything that is critical to you. Leave nothing out. The interview should flow easily and not feel like an interrogation. It won't, if done with ease of conversation and good planning.

Not all interviews will go the distance. If the person is unacceptable to you (i.e. terrible grooming habits, etc.), give an abbreviated interview. Ask a few questions and briefly explain your needs. View it as interview training! Tell the applicant you are interviewing others and will get back to them. Then be sure to call back in a day or two saying you've decided to hire someone else.

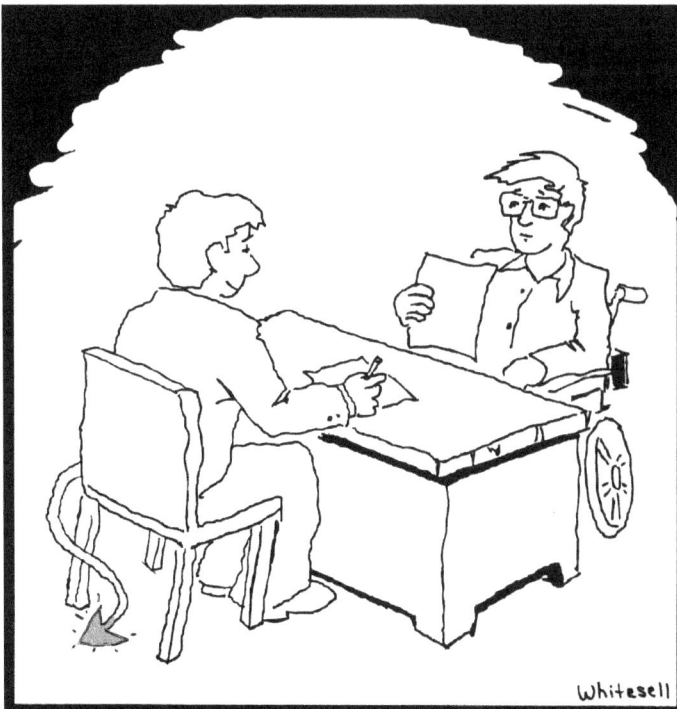

Whitesell

Sometimes, a single question can eliminate a prospect. Perhaps you failed to mention that you have a pet python or don't hire smokers. Perhaps the applicant says something to eliminate themselves (such as having a bad back). If you both agree the applicant is inappropriate for the position, apologize for the inconvenience and thank them for coming. However, don't close the door too quickly! Perhaps they have a friend who would be interested in the job. I also refer these applicants to other resources such as a Center for Independent Living as others may benefit from their offer to work.

Trust your instincts. If the applicant shows promise, continue with in-depth questions. If not, cut the interview short. If the applicant is not what you expected or if they start acting weird in the interview, calmly end the interview and show them to the door.

The final phase of a good interview is a tour of your home or apartment. Again, the key is to hear what they are telling you.

The prospective attendant's bedroom is often their primary interest as it will be their own space. If the bedroom is quite small, their response may be, "This is nicer than I thought it would be!" or, "Oh, dear. Where am I going to put all of my stuff in this little space?" Discuss their responses. Don't just say, "Well, this is the room! There's nothing I can do about it."

Are there ways you can compensate for problems? Some disabled employers offer their own bedroom (larger) to the live-in. Others allow the live-in to put some of their furnishings in the rest of the apartment (a TV or chair in the living room, for example). While some people bring little more than a few boxes of belongings, others bring all of their worldly possessions whether they need them or not. One live-in told me she just had to know that all of her things were nearby.

Discuss problems and hear concerns. It's the first step toward effective communication with a potential roommate and employee!

Chapter 7

Final Interviewing Phase

You've gone through a lengthy interview and the applicant shows great promise, but questions remain. How much do you really know about this person? The right questions will bring out hidden motives.

Some applicants will say anything to get the job. It is your task to be more cunning than they are — to catch lies, challenge inconsistencies, detect deception. This involves having a good ear... and more!

The "animal question" can help! In casual conversation (usually when the applicant is petting my cat or we are discussing pets), I ask if they ever thought of what animal they would be if they had the opportunity. I encourage them to respond. I give a positive response to their answer, no matter how strange, then ask why they made that choice. If they respond "a cat," I say, "I love cats! Why do you think you'd want to be a cat?" Even if they respond "a black widow spider," I say, "That's so interesting! Why a black widow spider?" Always show interest and enthusiasm. Their response reflects secrets of their soul!

Some responses I've gotten over the years proved astonishingly revealing:

- ♦ "A cat...because they just lay around all day and sleep." (In the interview, this applicant claimed to be a hard-worker who would have no problem getting me up at 6:30 a.m. Her response told me otherwise.)

- ♦ "A cat...because they look so innocent; no one would ever suspect them of doing anything evil." (This woman turned out to be concealing a drug and alcohol addiction, as well as a pregnancy!)

- ♦ "A dolphin...because I don't know enough about them and it would be interesting to see what it would be like to be one." (She never worked for a disabled person before. This told me she looked at the job as an interesting experience.)

- ♦ "A dog...because they command respect." (She did!)

- ♦ "A dog...because they are loyal and friendly." (She was.)

- ♦ "An eagle...because they are king of the sky and no other creature can control them." (This worker controlled the household and his disabled employer!)

It doesn't take a psychologist to interpret the responses to this question. What animal is selected means little. The reason it was selected means everything. Watch for key words or phrases in their response. This technique never fails. If you doubt it, ask your friends this question! The key is to be subtle. Don't say, "I can figure out the hidden you!"

Barbara Walters made a similar question keynote in her interviews when she asked what kind of tree people would want to be. Any object — what kind of car, for example — will do. The question is why the person wants to be that thing.

Make a list of interview questions so you can concentrate on what the applicant is saying.

Take time with the interview. Talk shop but also relax and chat about interests, current events or even the weather.

Do red flags surface? Does the person seem unusually nervous? Over-anxious to get the job? Bored? Impatient to leave? Do they keep coming back to money issues or how many days off they get? Are they guarded or secretive about their background? Do they seem obsessed with all of your "nice things"? Do they berate their past employers? Do they have a chip on their shoulder about life or how "everyone does them wrong"? Do they criticize former roommates, parents, family, girl/boyfriends? Some people are never happy and will surely make your life a living hell, as well.

The flip side is that the two of you really hit it off. Our tendency is to hold on to this person tightly, to lure them in fast. But as any angler knows, if you tug too hard on the line when you get a nibble, you'll surely lose the big ones.

Step back and give the applicant breathing space. You might say, "I don't know about you, but I really enjoyed meeting you today! I feel as though we're quite compatible and that this could work out well for both of us. I realize this is a big decision for you, however, so I want you to spend a little time thinking about it."

Suggest they come to see your care routine and return for training to see if the job is right for them. After that, have them work for you (for pay) to further see how you both feel.

I always tell applicants that I'm continuing to interview other people. This relieves pressure while letting the applicant know they must act quickly if they want the job. Far too often, they are indeed the only prospect though they never know it!

If you do have the luxury of having more than one applicant, tell your second choice you are in the process of training someone for the position though you are not sure if that person will take the job. Be careful not to be too glib with this second choice! They may end up being your only choice!!

Thank the applicant for coming, then set up a time they can return to witness your care routine. Ask them to confirm the day with you by phone before they come. This will help determine how responsible they are. If they fail to call or show as planned, give them a call. If they seem indecisive, don't push the issue. It may be their way of saying they are not interested. Accept this and move on.

Chapter 8

"It's Shhhow-time!"

Training is, without a doubt, the worst part of the PCA process. Like most people, I hate putting my fragile body into the hands of a stranger who may — or may not — do my care without hurting me. Transfers are the worst. Feeling their shaking arms around me, hearing a sigh or nervous laughter... I sometimes think I'm going to be sick.

Regardless of how uncomfortable it may be at the time, I realize that all of my wonderful veteran workers began as inexperienced trainees. I keep this in mind when the trainee rings the buzzer to announce her arrival. I take a deep breath, put on my happy face and say to myself, "It's shhhow-time!"

Regardless of how much time you spend describing your care plan, nothing can take the place of the first time the PCA applicant sees it first-hand.

Who should do the training? In my more "able" years, I relied on come-in PCAS morning and night. I'd interview someone, hand over the key to my apartment and say, "See you in the morning!" When they arrived, I talked them through my routine.

As my needs increased and my body became less resilient, I found it more and more difficult to talk someone through my care alone while tolerating the rigors of trial and error on my body. Instead, I began directing the training while having an experienced worker show the trainee what needed to be done.

The value of consumer-directed instruction helps the trainee focus on you as the one giving directives, not another worker. This establishes a redirection from the medical model to one that is consumer-directed which is especially

beneficial when training nursing assistants or others who worked in medical institutions, as these workers learn to only take direction from staff, not "patients."

As I further weakened, the trainee needed to watch longer before stepping in to do my care. Depending on the individual, I've learned to give more of the training control to the veteran worker. I consider each situation individually before determining who will direct the majority of training.

In the end, you must determine the best training method by considering:

- How good a trainer is the current PCA? Can you train better than they?

- Does the trainee come from an institution where you are referred to as "the patient"? If so, you should take the main lead in training.

- ♦ If the old and new workers are friends, you may want to let them work together at training.

- ♦ If your departing PCA is not good, train the new one yourself to break old habits or get a good back-up worker to help train.

Three tips for training:

1. Give a general overview of the procedure so the trainee knows what to expect.

2. Whenever possible, let the trainee observe the entire procedure the first time with general explanations. Realize they are probably intimidated, scared and over-whelmed, so going into specific detail at this point may be a waste of time.

3. Finally, determine what task or skill is most critical for you. In my case, it is whether of not they can physically lift me. Although other aspects of my care can be learned with time, if the person is not strong enough to lift me, nothing else matters. I encourage the trainee to attempt to lift me the first night to see if it's worth proceeding with training.

Don't rush training. This is critical to ensuring a good "find"!

Chapter 9

The Live-In Contract

You've decided to hire a particular individual for the position of live-in attendant. Although you've clearly voiced your expectations, you wonder if you might need more— a contract, perhaps?

A "contract" as seen here [See Appendix D] is not legally binding but does serve as a thorough, written document of expectations.

The following includes excerpts from my own contract. Going into detail will avoid future miscommunication.

My "Contract in Good Faith" begins, "We are about to enter into a unique working and living arrangement. The intent of this contract is to clarify the rights, responsibilities and expectations of this arrangement." The document should be viewed as a helpful tool for both parties.

My care:

Describe your general care, hours the PCA is on and off duty, and so on.

Other duties:

List additional responsibilities: i.e. shopping, cleaning, cooking, banking, driving, pet care, etc., as well as what they are not responsible for!

Your employer:

If your funding comes from a source other than you (i.e. government, agency, private insurance), state who the employer is. For me, even though the funding comes from a state and county source, I technically remain the employer. The worker will need to know this for future references.

Pay:

Explain the pay rate and how this is determined. Are they paid by the hour or given a salary? Do you control the rate they receive or does a funding source? Who draws the checks, and when? If the checks come from an outside source and arrive late, are you responsible for loaning the worker money?

Let the worker know when they will not be paid. For me, these include:

♦ When I am in the hospital

♦ When I am on vacation (unless they come along as my caregiver)

♦ When someone else works in their place

♦ When they take time off

Let them know if you offer paid vacations or paid medical leave or if they have a right to unemployment compensation.

Cleaning:

Spell out their daily cleaning responsibilities or if you hire outside help for this. Remember, everyone's concept of "clean" is different. Do you expect your PCA to vacuum once a month? Scrub the floors on their hands and knees? Move furniture to clean? Be specific!

Time off:

How much? When? Are dates flexible? I include the clause, "You may waive time off, if you wish; however, I have the right to require you to take time off if I feel it is in our mutual interest or to benefit your physical or mental health." I find some workers have more interest in their paycheck than in my safety so may refuse time off even if they have a bad back or other problems. This clause allows me to dictate time off.

Contracting out for care:

Who is responsible for finding your respite care workers? If your PCA wants time off and finds a replacement worker for you, is that acceptable? Or do you or an agency provide workers? What if the respite worker cancels or another can't be found? Do you have emergency back-ups (such as family) or must the live-in waive their day off?

Personal property:

I include: "I assume full responsibility for any damage I personally do to your property through accident or negligence. I will not assume responsibility for any damage to your property caused by my cat. A closed bedroom door will prohibit her from entering if you choose for her to stay out... You have a right to put a keyed lock on your bedroom door; however, management must be given a copy of the key... I will respect your property and never enter your room or peruse your property without permission. I expect the same from you."

Their room:

What rights do/don't they have? Can they decorate? Paint the walls? Hang heavy objects? Burn candles? I include rules regarding insect problems, property damage and the need for yearly inspections by management.

Mail, phone, TV:

Who retrieves the mail and where is it left? Can/must the live-in get their own phone line? Is cable TV an option?

Kitchen procedures:

Can your live-in use your pots, pans, dishes, flatware, appliances, etc.? Must they provide their own? You may have an expensive Teflon pan that can be irreparably damaged with one wrong use, fine glassware that can be broken, and flatware that can be lost. By specifying what is available for their use, you will save aggravation and dollars down the road. I also require that "All grains, flour, sugar and so forth must be kept in sealed, glass jars — no bags or boxes — to avoid insect infestation."

Garbage disposal:

Yes, I go so far as to explain what can and can not be put down the garbage disposal! This has saved me many costly repairs.

Refrigerator/food:

Determine your food/eating/grocery arrangement. Options might include: providing all the food and groceries; splitting this expense; sharing some food or meals while splitting others; or keeping food completely separate. The Great Refrigerator Debate can be grounds for roommate "divorce" and should not be taken lightly. Spell out all specifics in a contract!

Bathroom rules:

These might include where to put wet towels, if you need the seat to be left up or down, or any other needs or quirks.

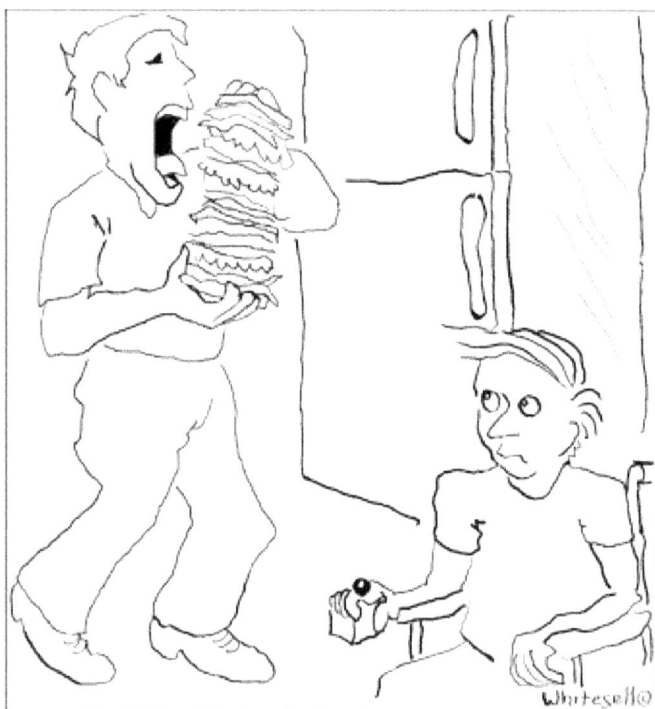

The Great Refrigerator Debate can be grounds for roommate "divorce"...

Universal precautions:

It is essential you make latex/vinyl gloves, masks and any other protection available to all workers. If they choose not to use these and you don't mind if they don't, it's up to the both of you. But you must make this protection available. Disposal of used items must be done appropriately; e.g. gloves rolled off cuff to fingers, turning the contaminated gloves inside out. Keep anti-bacterial soap at the sink as well. Appropriately dispose of syringes, adult diapers and other such items.

I provide/they provide:

I include: "I will provide paper towels and toilet paper for normal use. You provide your own Kleenex and other paper products for other use (i.e. paper towels used to clean your car, etc.). You will pay toward toilet paper if you regularly use it instead of facial tissue... You provide all supplies for personal use including light bulbs for your room, office/school supplies, kitchen supplies and so forth. You are welcome to use my cleaning products and vacuum to clean your room whenever you wish... You are expected to turn off all lights, fans, TV, etc., in your room before leaving for extended hours. Windows should not be opened more than a crack on cold days to avoid excessive heating bills." These things may seem picky until they become constant irritations or costly problems!

Vehicle use:

If you own a vehicle, spell out your rules regarding driving it (with or without you). Be firm, and don't renege later if you decide your vehicle is off limits to them even if they argue they need it "just this once"!

Overnight guests:

Spell out rules involving boy/girlfriends, family, children and others spending the night as well as how many people can stay per night, where they sleep, and if you require prior notice.

Smoking/alcohol/drugs:

Spell out your rules loud and clear on each **topic!**

Police record:

Although I mention this in the interview, I reiterate it in the contract: "I may run a police check on you and reserve the right to fire or not hire you based on the results."

Grounds for dismissal:

Develop your criteria for dismissal and hold firm to it! Mine includes:

♦ Gross negligence of job responsibilities.

♦ Police record which I deem unacceptable.

♦ Possession or use of illicit drugs by you or your guests.

♦ Working while intoxicated.

♦ Theft of any type or degree.

♦ Unauthorized use of my van.

♦ Physical or verbal abuse toward myself or my animals.

♦ Unreported pregnancy.

♦ Blatant lies and deception.

♦ Actions which result in warnings from management.

Dismissal/resignation:

Most state laws do not require you to give any notice when firing a live-in PCA as they are not sharing rent (unless this is your arrangement). Instead, free rent is a perk, much as it is for nannies or house-keepers.

Forwarding of mail:

Make sure you have a permanent address to forward mail. Keep in mind you can forward mail or return it, but it is a federal crime to dispose of first class mail.

Management rules:

In my lease, the wrongful actions of my live-in PCA may lead to my eviction. I specify all management rules which affect us both!

Above and beyond...

I conclude my contract with, "Above and beyond all of the aforementioned, it is imperative we show each other respect, courtesy, dignity and honesty. Without these, none of the above matters."

Both you and the live-in should sign and date the contract and each keep a copy.

The reason for having a contract is to create a sound foundation for good communication by putting the rules and expectations in writing. Ambiguity, poor communication and lack of authority are some of the biggest reasons for failure of these working relationships.

Chapter 10

"Say, What?"

Communication is the key to any good relationship, be it business, romance or social. It can be the single most important component in making or breaking your relationship with a Personal Care Attendant (PCA). Sadly, you can only control one-half of the communication process, but this is better than no control at all.

One disabled neighbor came to me with a problem. "You have a lot of experience with workers," he said, "What's the best way to go about firing one?" I asked what his particular situation involved. "It's my cleaning lady," he said. "She's doing a lousy job." "What do you mean, exactly?" I asked. "She doesn't move things out of the kitchen before she mops the floor," he said, adding, "She doesn't lift things off of shelves before she dusts. Things like that."

"Well," I prodded, "what happens when you tell her that's not how you want it done?" "Oh," he quickly responded, "I've never told her! She's a cleaning lady! She's supposed to know these things!"

People aren't mind readers. If you want something, you need to ask for it.

In my family, we were told things like, "You shouldn't have to be told to (clean up your room, do your homework, pick up your dirty clothes, etc.). You should just be able to see that it needs to be done!" Although that may be true in a perfect world, we don't live in such a place! Instead, we must be clear and direct if we want our needs met.

If you want the garbage taken out don't say, "Boy, that kitchen garbage sure does fill up fast," as this may leave you with little more than an acknowledgment from a PCA: "Yep, it sure does!"

Instead, be specific with your request: "Please take out the kitchen garbage when you leave." Follow up as they are leaving: "Did you remember the garbage?" **Take responsibility for tasks needing to be done**. Don't expect your PCA to do it all automatically.

Determine how best to communicate with your PCA. Some people have a terrific memory; others need reminders. I had one live-in who said I should make a list to remind her of tasks. So everyday I made lists, and everyday the tasks were completed.

When the next live-in PCA moved in, I made her lists as well. After a few days, she became irate and said, "Why do you insult me with all these lists? Don't you think I can remember to do things when you ask?" (Her memory, as it turned out, was uncanny.)

58

ASK how your PCA wants to be reminded of tasks.

We get angry when things aren't done right. "I told her to put it in the bedroom!" Is that really what you said? Or did you say, "Put it in the other room"? Our directions are often vague. "The other room... the dresser... the shelf." We need to be specific.

Failure to be understood is the fault of the speaker. Work to ensure the listener hears your words and understands your intent. The primary responsibility for this is yours, not theirs.

We are poor listeners. We tend to be thinking about other things and not concentrating on listening. Keep this in mind when you give someone instructions.

Better communication can be aided by employing common courtesy. A written reminder that you will be late on Tuesday, adding please and thank you to your requests, asking (not telling) a worker to do a special task are all simple acts of courtesy which can make work nicer for the both of you.

Chapter 11

Neither a Borrower, Nor a Lender Be

It all seems straight-forward enough: a home health aide comes in, introduces herself and asks what needs to be done. She is the employee; you are the employer. But the line that separates the two can become fuzzy at times, downright absent at others.

Sometimes the employer and employee become friends. But is there an easy way to remain friendly while keeping a working relationship? And how does one create a homey work setting without being taken advantage of?

Once when I was in the bathtub, a come-in PCA burst into the bathroom, looked in the mirror and rubbed her lips together. "What do you think of this lipstick?" she asked. "Fine," I responded, still a bit shocked she'd barge in on my privacy like this. "Did you just buy it?" I asked. "Oh, no," she proudly announced. "It's yours! I saw it on your vanity so I decided to try it!"

Clearly, she saw nothing wrong with this. In her experience, this might just be the way she gets by — using, taking, borrowing from others. **What is normal, after all, is what we experience in our own life.**

This does not mean we have to accept their behavior in our home! It is up to us to set the standards while they are under our roof. Don't shout or scream or call them names. Just present your house rules in a clear and concise manner: "Could you please take your boots off at the door? The wet snow will dirty the floor." You may have to repeat the message. Don't be harsh; just remind them.

Clear, consistent rules will make life easier for everyone. This goes just as well for wet boots as for food and finances — two relationship stumbling blocks.

Food –

Is there is a sign hanging on your refrigerator door which reads, "Free food"? Some workers seem to act as if there is! They open the door and help themselves to food or drinks without even asking! Others beg, saying they are so thirsty or so hungry... Could they just have one? If you say "No," does the worker help themselves, anyway?

To stop this from happening, determine in advance what you're willing to offer, then remain firm on your rules. Some options might include that:

♦ The worker can store food or drink in your refrigerator for break time.

♦ They can buy soda from you if you have extra (and if they have the cash!).

♦ They must always ask but never just help themselves.

- They can help themselves to whatever you have.

- They can share any meal they make for you.

- If they buy their own food, they can eat with you.

- They are not to eat or drink while on duty.

- They can help themselves to water but nothing else.

Be sure to make the rules clear from the onset and remain firm:

"Did you just take that Pepsi from the 'frig?"

"Yes, but it's so hot, and I'm dying of thirst!"

"I know it's hot. Drink as much water as you'd like, but I told you before, I don't want you drinking my Pepsi. It's hard for me to get it from the store, and soda is expensive. Please don't take my Pepsi anymore."

Don't accept excuses like, "I left my soda at home" or "I forgot my money." When it comes to drink, offer water. If they say they don't like water, they must not be too thirsty.

Neither a Borrower, Nor a Lender Be

Or, "That's not mine. It belongs to my roommate. Please don't take it anymore."

Or, "There's a soda machine downstairs. Please don't drink my supply."

Never offer alcoholic beverages during work hours. You put their job and your safety in jeopardy.

Money —

Isn't it odd: We are often the ones on a fixed income, yet they are the ones who continually borrow money from us!

> "Could I just borrow a dollar for bus fare to get home?"

> "I have no rain coat. Could I borrow $10 for a cab?"

> "My ol' man beat me and took my check so he could buy drugs! Could I just have a twenty till pay day?"

Rest assured, you're not the only sucker in town. They find all of us in time!

The issue of borrowing money is going to come up, so decide now what your policy will be. It may differ from one PCA to the next.

♦ If you lend money, ask when it will be repaid. When that day comes, ask for your money if it is not offered. Be firm.

♦ Never lend more money if you have not been repaid from the previous time.

♦ Write down the amount loaned, the date, and when it will be repaid.

♦ Think of lending cash as gambling: never give out more than you can afford to lose. Even the best workers quit, get fired or skip town.

- Never let ANYONE see how much money you have on hand! "Can I borrow a five?" can turn into "...a couple twenties?" if they see you have it!

- Never feel pressured into lending money to anyone, no matter how sad the story or nice the person is. If you don't want to lend it or can't afford to do so, DON'T!

We all run short of cash from time to time, but be aware of the worker who is always "short."

It's difficult not to lend money to the person who has just gotten you dressed, bathed and toileted. Perhaps we feel we owe them this gesture. But keep in mind they are paid to help us. We don't feel obligated to lend money to our mail carrier, physician or the maintenance man. Yet these people also perform valuable functions for us. The PCA will always find someone to lend money. That "someone" need not be you!

Chapter 12

Sex, Drugs and PCAs!

I noted some common stumbling blocks that blur the roles of employer   and employee such as food and money issues. But the line betweenthe two is totally erased when taken to the next level: sex and drugs.

Jack, an attractive quadriplegic, hired Brenda, an agency home health aide, who was divorced with three small children. After getting to know him, Brenda asked if it was okay to bring her kids to work as she had no sitter. "Sure, this one time" led to a second — and a third. Soon, she began leaving the children with him when she ran errands. When she came without the kids, she claimed to have a migraine and would sleep on his couch the entire work time.

> Just when his tolerance for her antics had about reached its limit, she further dirtied the waters by sleeping with him. After that, he was so entrenched in the mire, he was incapable of being an "employer" — or of getting his work needs met.

In another situation, Willie was a heavy drug user. In no time, he and his home health aide were smoking marijuana together — during work hours, of course. The aide soon bought drugs from Willie, promising to pay him when her check came in two weeks. Pay day came and went, but Willie was never reimbursed for the dope he continued to supply. "I swear, I'll pay you next time!" she said, though never did. In time, Willie found himself stuck with a useless worker whom he could not fire because of money still owed nor could he report her due to his contribution to the illegal activities!

Scott, a newly-disabled quad, turned down my referral of a qualified male live-in saying he was holding out for a female as he wanted to find a girlfriend who liked to "party." He hired Jenny who soon divulged she had a boyfriend. In time the boyfriend, a heavy cocaine user, moved in as well. Jenny got fed up with the boyfriend and moved out, but the ex-boyfriend became hostile and refused to leave. Scott soon became a prisoner of his own apartment, afraid to leave for fear this guy would sell his property to buy more coke. In the end, Scott was almost evicted because of the actions of the coke-addict "roommate." He also never got a girlfriend as he had hoped.

In the business world, there are strict rules which prohibit fraternization between employer and employee yet we often ignore these same rules in our own work setting. It is important we develop personal guidelines in dealing with PCAS.

♦ Be up front with workers who want to cross the line when it comes to sex and drugs. "Just say no!" is not bad advice!

- If you choose to get high or drink, wait until the worker has left. If you need help in accomplishing either, refrain from asking an agency worker; instead, rely on a friend or willing live-in.

- Don't partake in sexual activities with your employees. If you can't "just say no," socialize during non-work hours. Sadly, you may discover that your worker's romantic interest may languish when they are no longer getting paid to spend time with you.

- Don't plot to make a PCA your girl or boyfriend. It can only end up in a disaster.

- Don't encourage your PCA to participate in illicit or sexual activities.

Simply, you can be friendly, develop a warm and trusting relationship, have fun and be comfortable with your workers without getting high or going to bed with them.

Chapter 13

Perks for Live-Ins

Finding and training a live-in PCA is only the beginning of your work. Keeping them is the real task! The following are some perks to entice your PCA into staying longer and remaining happier!

A live-in attendant has the right to expect:

♦ a clear and concise job description;

♦ wages paid in full and on time;

♦ sufficient time off;

♦ a private room/area of their own;

♦ to be treated with dignity and respect.

Unfortunately, most PCA positions are long on hours and low on pay. But "perks" — those little extras you are not obligated to provide — can often make a big difference in a worker's job contentment. The following are examples of perks.

A place to live —

From splitting the rent to granting free room and board plus pay, offers vary depending on the extent of care needed, space and income available.

> Cindy offered no pay while expecting a
> live-in attendant to do extensive personal

care from early morning until late night. She also expected this worker to split the rent. Not surprisingly, she had few responses to her ads.

Use common sense when considering what to request or offer. No one will work for free and pay rent!

Utilities —

Free gas/electric, water, heat and air conditioning are major perks for anyone who has paid for their own in the past!

Phone/TV/cable —

It is wise not to share your phone line. Instead, you may offer to pay installation charges for a second line in their room giving them the option to connect the service (at their expense).

Even if your live-in has their own phone, save yourself headaches — and possibly hundreds of dollars in phone bills — by putting a block put on your line for:

- ♦ "900/976" calls;
- ♦ all international calls; or,
- ♦ all long distance calls, excluding toll-free or those made with calling cards.

There is usually no fee to initiate the block.

Cable TV is a big perk to many! But the question is whose TV has cable? If it is on your TV, you may find your couch potato roommate has sprouted roots in your living room! If you don't mind (or even enjoy) their company, fine. But remember you are paying for the service. Don't be intimidated into watching what (or when) you don't want.

A better option may be to install a cable hook-up in their room (your expense) and let them initiate the service. I charge my live-ins $10/month to cover the cost of leasing the second converter box and remote control in addition to paying toward the cable bill.

Most cable stations offer a pay-per-view option for films, concerts, wrestling and special events. A phone call automatically orders the showing. Most offer an option to require a Personal Identification Number (PIN) to activate the connection. You would be wise to have this. If your roommate wants to order a film or event, you order it. Never give out your PIN number! As special events can easily run $50 each, consider requiring payment in advance before ordering.

It's all too common for kind-hearted disabled employers to be left with enormous telephone and cable bills when workers "blow out of Dodge" leaving us holding the bag... of bills!

Food —
It's no secret you can eat better and more economically splitting the food bill. The secret to this

success is to discuss your buying/eating habits in detail beforehand. Some questions to ask include:

- How many meals do you each eat at home daily?
- What do you normally eat?
- In what quantities?
- Are you a bargain shopper or a binge buyer?
- Are generic brands acceptable or do you insist on expensive brand names?
- What costs are to be split: cigarettes and beer, or just food?
- Do you eat leftovers or toss what is not used that day?

One alternative is to have separate refrigerator shelves. This leaves little question as to whose food and drink is whose. Make sure guests or other workers don't help themselves to that which belongs to the other person.

A place to live —

Often, the commodity in shortest supply is space. Unless you own a home, your roommate will be lucky to get little more than their own bedroom. Some of us barely have enough room for our own things much less someone else's. Still, space must be provided. At a minimum, a live-in needs their own room and storage in the bathroom and kitchen. If there is a locker, consider sharing this as well.

How much each person brings varies considerably. Generally, college students are used to sharing a small dorm room so have few possessions. Someone who has lived on their own may have furniture and more. Identify all available space in the interview.

In some cases, it is the *disabled* individual who has little more than a bedroom full of possession. This allows the live-in to furnish the apartment with their own belongings.

Similarly, some disabled individuals allow their live-in to have the larger bedroom. A smaller room is harder to negotiate by wheelchair, so don't switch unless you're sure it will work for you. Remember, you're paying the rent!

Transportation —
For live-ins who don't have a car, it can be a chore to take the bus to get groceries or run errands. If you have a vehicle, you may consider granting limited use to your live-in. Consider their age and driving record in making this decision. Set limits! Can they only borrow the vehicle to run errands for you? For short jaunts of their own? To get to/from a part-time job? Or anytime they want?

Use of your vehicle is a wonderful gesture, but your misjudgment can mean the end of your transportation and/or insurance. If you do not want your live-in to touch your vehicle, keep the keys on your person and ask neighbors to advise you, immediately, if they witness the live-in driving off.

A nice live-in of my neighbor John got drunk one night, took John's van and went on a 70-mile, hit-and-run rampage before being stopped by the state patrol.

This live-in said hi to me before leaving. He was carrying a paper bag containing what I believed to be alcohol. As I watched him drive off, I thought how foolish of John to allow this guy to take his van!

You set the tone for the living and working relationship. Friendly or professional, warm or aloof, your live-in will no doubt respond to the mood

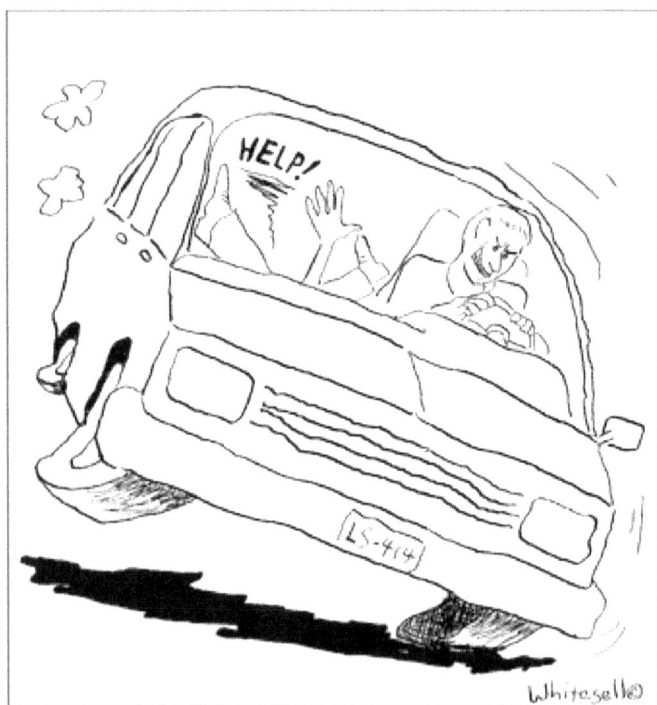

Transportation — set limits!

you've created

As it turned out, John never told any of us the van was strictly off limits to the live-in nor that the live-in was a recovering alcoholic!

The little things —

The "little things" can add up to big things over time. Allowing a live-in's friend to spend the night, being flexible with your schedule and time off, treating them to an occasional meal or movie, being a good listener, letting them know in advance if you will be home late so they can make other plans — all make living together more "livable."

Chapter 14

The "Live-Out" Live-In

We all know how safe and secure it feels to have that one special person to help us with all our daily needs. For many, that is (or was) Mom. For some, a devoted spouse. For others, a rare caregiver. Sometime circumstance dictates that this person be the only one who can--or will--do the care. Although not always healthy, it is simply the way it is.

In most cases, however, there is a choice of who works for us; yet many disabled individuals expect--even demand--one person be there for all of their needs working "24/7." Little do they know, this is a recipe for failure.

The number one reason good care goes bad is caregiver burnout. Without ample time for their own needs, a caregiver cannot care for our needs... or at least, without sacrificing health or sanity (theirs and ours). We'd benefit from dividing long work hours between as many workers as possible. My own experience shows this can work extremely well.

A year ago, I was having a difficult time finding a replacement for my live-in PCA. When I decided to change my ad from seeking "one live-in caregiver" to "people to work one or more nights per week," I was inundated with responses! Three girls now share my weekly work schedule. Here's how it works:

Three girls share a furnished bedroom. Each is given a dresser drawer and closet space. The girls bring their own bedding (sheets/blankets or sleeping bag) as well as items to share in the room including a TV, VCR, lamps, alarm clock, plants, and decorations. (You could provide these yourself.) I provide cable TV connection.

I invite them to a dinner (pizza or sub sandwiches) where they meet as soon as all are hired. Although they will never work at the same time, they will be functioning as a team with my care. I disseminate work schedules and each other's phone numbers. They are encouraged to make their own subsequent work schedules and to trade work days with each other as they want or need.

I keep the master work schedule posted in my bedroom where all changes MUST be written. If conflicts occur, the person's name that appears on my master will be held accountable. In over a year, I have never had even one conflict or problem. This system has given the girls tremendous autonomy and flexibility.

My goal is to have someone here every night to do my care. As long as that goal is met, it is in everyone's best interest that I remain as flexible as possible in letting them work out whatever schedule they wish. Of course, I still dictate times and make special requests as needed.

Wouldn't it be easier on me to have the same person working every night? *Of course!* Don't I prefer one workers over another? *You bet!* Isn't it confusing to have different people every night? *Boy, I'll say!*

But, with that said, this is still the best system I've ever had.

- ♦ No longer do I worry what I'll do when someone gets sick or leaves, as there is now a TEAM to help pick up the slack if one member is unable to work.

- ♦ No longer do I worry about whether or not someone is being worked too much or too little, as *she* calls the shots on when she works and when she doesn't.

- ♦ No longer do I worry what I'll do if *I* get sick and need extra help, as there are *several* people who care for me... and care about me!

- ♦ As a plus, there is the joy of such varied personalities in my life every day. Variety *truly is* the spice of life!

My only dilemma is how to answer when I'm asked if I have a "live-in attendant." But I now answer, "Well, sort of. I have 'live-out' live-ins! And it's working *beautifully*, thank you!"

Chapter 15

The Consumer's Responsibility

Although this book is about "attendants from Hell," there is no question there are more than a few "consumers from Hell" to go around! Clearly, many working relationships are doomed the minute the PCA walks in the door. We can't blame all of our problems on the workers; we must assume some of the responsibility ourselves.

There are daily responsibilities to living on your own. You must either learn to do these things yourself or delegate them to others. Keep in mind, if you can't articulate your needs, you will get just that: nothing!

Unfortunately, a number of workers will do as little work as possible. Unless you instruct them as to what to do, how to do it and when, a task may never get done (or done the way you want).

So the first task is to figure out what you want or need and when things must be done. For example: how often do you want to shower? Whose responsibility will it be to shower you? How long will the procedure take? What time of day is it to be done? How much can you do for yourself? All this for a simple shower! But these are necessary questions to answer before you can instruct someone else to help you.

Go down the list: medications, meal planning, grocery shopping, laundry duties, house cleaning and so on. If need be, have someone write everything in a notebook for you regarding each. Give a copy to each worker, then hold them accountable to the tasks.

Does your apartment resemble a war zone? The apartments of many disabled individuals often do. Dirty dishes stacked in the sink; trash overflowing; laundry piled up; floors sticky with grit and grime; medication bottles left open with pills spilt on the floor; defrosted hamburger meat in a bloody pool dripping from counter to floor. I've seen these horrors more than once.

Whose fault is this? YOURS! YOU are the employer! It is your responsibility to make sure daily tasks get done. Yes, in a perfect world the worker would automatically do these things. But, as we've learned, we don't live in a perfect world.

The problem becomes self-perpetuating. The worker tries to get by with as little work as possible; you ignore it; your home begins to look and smell like a pig sty; no one likes living in a pig sty; the mess builds to insurmountable proportions; they quit because they hate living there.

This is your home. If you can't take responsibility for ensuring a clean, pleasant living (and working) environment, you may be better off in another type of living situation where someone else takes over these tasks. As stated in the beginning of this book, **independent living is not for everyone.**

Here are some of your responsibilities to a live-in PCA:

- **Establish a definitive job description and stick to it.**

    Determine (mutually or by yourself) job duties as well as a time frame in which tasks must be completed. Make sure the PCA agrees to these. Then, enforce the agreement.

- **Provide your live-in with personal time and space.**

    Most live-ins say it's difficult, after a while, to live where they work. Although they physically may be unable to get away from work, we can make it possible for them to get away, psychologically, by providing them private time and personal space.

- **Make sure they get paid on time.**

    Most people live from paycheck to paycheck. If time sheets must be submitted, make sure they are done so on time. When their paycheck arrives, make sure they get it immediately.

- **Moderate disputes between workers.**

    Sometimes live-in and come-in workers butt heads regarding how a job is being — or not being — done. It is your responsibility, as the employer, to rectify these differences and manage each worker.

- **Give the worker ample time off.**

"All work and no play makes Jack a dull boy." It also makes PCAS up and quit! Negotiate time off needs with your workers.

- **RESPECT your worker!**

This person is your employee not your hand-maiden or subordinate. "Please," "thank you," and other common courtesies go a long way in keeping a worker longer.

Frequently, someone seeking work as a live-in asks if I know of an available position. Sadly, I often say, "Yes, but you wouldn't want to work for him." My response never has to do with the extent of an individual's care but, instead, of the deplorable living and working conditions. "Her apartment reeks." "He does drugs." "He has scary friends."

If you want good workers, you must provide a good living and working environment.

Chapter 16

The PCA's Responsibility

Consumers aren't the only ones who need tips; PCAS do, too Whether applying to work part-time or especially to live in with a disabled individual, you — as a Personal Care Attendant — need to do your own interviewing!

It goes without saying, you need to understand your job duties, pay, time off and living arrangement. But make sure you clearly understand these things!

- **Are you the only worker or will others share duties?**

  Do you have specific times off when another worker is on duty? If that worker fails to show, are you obligated to work their shift?

- **Are you expected to perform care outside the home?**

  Must you meet the disabled individual at school or work for their care or accompany them shopping or to social events? If they spend the night at a friend's house, are you expected to run over to do their care?

- **What does "day off" really mean?**
  What hours are you off? Are you expected to do any work during those hours? Must you leave the premises or can you stay?

The following tips may further help you get the information you need to have a successful working and living relationship.

Ask questions. We won't bite. If you don't ask, you won't know. Chances are you will be nervous in the interview, so write down questions ahead of time. Here are some you may want to ask:

- **"What is your disability?"**
  We're used to people stumbling to find the right words. "Ah, how did you get like that? Err, I mean, what's wrong with you? Well, I meant..." It's okay; we get it.. "May I ask the nature of your disability?" is the proper question, but "What is your disability?" is just fine. If you are unfamiliar with a particular disease or disability, ask about it. It will help you better understand our needs.

- **"How long have you been living on your own?"**
  This will give you an idea of how established we are at managing our care. Your experience as a live-in will differ tremendously depending if you are the first or tenth live-in for the individual.

- **"How many live-ins have you had in that time?"**

If someone runs through several live-ins a year, don't think you will be the one who will last. There is usually a reason for the many turn-overs. Find out what it is.

- **"Tell me about your former live-ins!"**

Beware of consumers who bad-mouths every live-in employee they ever had! You will surely be next, whether you deserve it or not!

- **"Tell me about your relationship with your family?"**

This will help you understand if the family can be viewed as a support in their independent living process.

- **"What happens if I get sick?"**

Who does their care in this situation? Make sure the answer is someone other than yourself!

- **Sex, drugs and rock 'n' roll.**

What kind of situation can't you live with? Find out their religious belief (or lack thereof) if this makes a difference to you. Are you/they a day or night person? Is sexual preference an issue with either of you? Do you/they use drugs or alcohol? Do you/they prefer classical music or rap? Can your boy/girlfriend spend the night? Do you mind if their boy/girlfriend spends the night? Ask what your responsibilities will be on those evenings. Will their partner do their care? Are you expected to help their partner if they are also disabled? Don't be afraid to ask!

- **Animal kingdom.**

  Ask if you will be living with a pet and what the extent of your pet responsibilities will be. Make sure you meet the critter!

Most of all, BE HONEST! I've had live-ins conceal bad backs, pregnancy, drug and alcohol addiction and clinical depression. You may end up with the job, but you won't have it for long. I've given up trying to cover all the bases in the interview knowing I will always miss something.

> Tara was an ambitious 19-year-old. Although she could barely lift me, she kept saying she would improve with practice. I knew she wouldn't work out, yet I didn't want to squelch her enthusiasm.
>
> The following day she called me to say she forgot to mention she had this problem where she passes out without warning! I couldn't believe it! She said it's brought on by stress. I said, "So, what you're saying is that if you're trying to lift me and become nervous, you may pass out with me in your arms?" "Yes," she said, "I guess I might."
>
> Needless to say, we didn't continue training. But the point is, what if we had? We'd both have suffered severely from this one "oversight."

Without a doubt, working as a live-in Personal Care Attendant can be a nice way of getting a place to live and a nice salary for relatively short work hours. Each live-in arrangement differs. Some require "24/7" care. These situations, however, are

90

less common. Increasingly, work hours and duties are shared by a combination of workers and funding sources. Find out what your specific duties will — and won't — be. Don't be afraid to ask about specifics!

If you get the job, keep the lines of communication open. It should go without saying, you need to discuss your needs and problems with your employer.

When you decide to quit, give as much notice as possible. Leaving a disabled individual without care borders on being inhumane. I have personally known of folks who have spent days sleeping in their wheelchair with a pillow on a dresser, been left on a couch with no means of calling for help, and been forced to move into a nursing home when a worker walks out with little or no notice. Many of us require months to find a replacement. At the very least, provide a one-month notice.

Chapter 17

The Real ER!

Television portrays the hospital emergency room as an exciting — even sexy — place to be. But as anyone who's ever been in one knows, this is far from the reality, a fact especially true for people with physical disabilities.

Yet, if we must seek emergency medical care, we'd better be able to express our needs — even if we're unconscious — if we expect to survive the experience.

Your health care is your responsibility once you move out on your own. This means you must have a thorough understanding of your medical condition and be able to direct others as to the best way to meet your needs.

Know your medications —

Be it prescription drugs or over-the-counter products, medication is crucial in keeping most of us healthier and more comfortable. But sometimes the vast array of orange, plastic pill containers seem to take on a life of its own. It's hard to keep them all straight. Do I take two green pills at three? Or three blue pills at two? And when did I last take the yellow ones?

Working together, you and your PCA can keep everything straight.

♦ **Explain your medication.** Most of your personal care workers are curious about what medications you take. Help them understand by saying, "If you're interested, I'll be glad to tell you what these pills are for." I explain this even though I do not need assistance in taking them. Even if you feel this is a private issue, you can still offer general explanations. "The pills I take help my spasms," "This medication is important to reduce my pain," or "I have a bladder problem which this medicine keeps under control."

♦ **Make a list of your medications and when they are to be taken.** Post it where your workers can find it. This is critical if you need help taking them or if you ever need hospitalization. You may want to describe the appearance of the pill along with the name, i.e. "red and white horse pills."

♦ **Clearly label bottles.** Don't re-use old bottles until the label is rubbed off or place pills in unmarked pill organizers if at all possible. If you must place them in organizers, keep the original bottles nearby so emergency medical personnel can identify which pills are which.

♦ **Keep medications in one or two areas.** Don't have them scattered throughout several rooms. Keep prescription medications within sight for workers and paramedics to easily find if an emergency were to arise.

♦ **Do you need help taking medication?** A missed pill could mean trouble. A dropped pill could mean death or illness to the child or pet who finds it. All this and child-proof bottles, too!

As a Shaklee distributor, I sold vitamins to several elderly people in the apartment complex where I once lived. As child-proof caps are impossible for me to open, I asked one arthritic customer how she managed. In a very matter-of-fact manner, she said she took her hammer and shattered the plastic bottles, picked out the vitamins and threw away the broken pieces! I was stunned she had never mentioned this in the couple years she regularly bought from me!

The problem was rectified by my asking the gentleman who brought the vitamins to open her bottle when he delivered it to her. She was forever grateful.

♦ **Make pill taking easier.** Upon request, prescriptions can be put in twist-open containers (not child-proof). Many pills are also available in liquid form (ask your doctor). Pill crushers and pill splitters are available at pharmacies and health stores if this is a need.

- **Never give others your medication!** Although our large array of pills is sometimes a tempting sight to workers and friends, never give medication to others under any circumstances. The warning on pill bottles — "Federal law prohibits use by any other person" — means just that: it is a federal crime to let other people take your prescriptions. Although stool softeners may not be a highly sought after drug, others are. The following are but a few drugs workers and others may try to get from you:

Narcotic containing painkillers:

Percocet, Percodan, Darvon, Demerol, Fiorinal, Vicodin and medication containing codeine or morphine

Tranquilizers/antidepressants:

Librium, Valium, Dalmane, Serax, Elavil

Helpful Medical Documents —

Written information prepared in advance can save your life, but most is useless if you are the only one who knows about it! The following are some documents which can be invaluable when medical emergencies arise. Discuss each one with your physicians, family and primary caregivers.

- **Emergency Medical Information** [Appendix E]. This is a list identifying your medical condition, history, medications and so on.

Keep it where others — especially workers and paramedics — can easily find it. This should include everything a hospital emergency room would need to know about your existing condition. Modify the sample list to reflect your particular situation. Update it regularly.

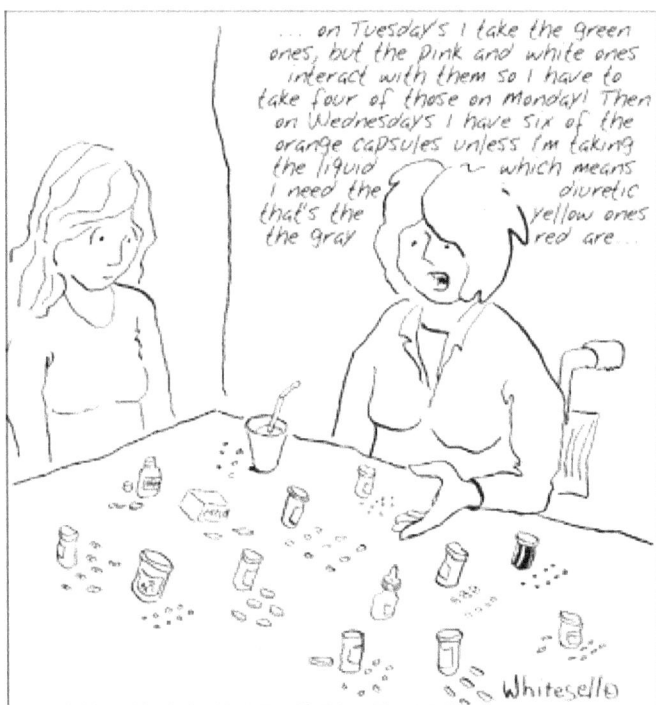

... on Tuesdays I take the green ones, but the pink and white ones interact with them so I have to take four of those on Mondays! Then on Wednesdays I have six of the orange capsules unless I'm taking the liquid ~ which means I need the diuretic that's the yellow ones the gray red are ...

Whiteselle

Explain your medication.

♦ **Living Will.** This one-page document identifies your intent regarding artificial support if you are terminally ill or, in some states, in a persistent vegetative state. Simply, this document lets others know whether or not you want to refuse treatments which would "merely prolong the process of dying." A strict set of medical criteria must be met before your Living Will would take effect. Sources for obtaining this free form (which requires no legal assistance or filing fee) include legal aid departments and your state legislators. Send copies to your physicians and family. Keep the original.

♦ **Durable Power of Attorney for Health Care** is a critical piece of legislation that allows you to designate two people to make decisions on your behalf in the event you are unable to do so. This is more flexible and comprehensive than the Living Will and applies to all situations in which the person is incapable of making decisions, not just when terminally ill. These designees can access your medical records, speak to your doctor, and decide if certain procedures should be implemented or discontinued based on your interests. It is a powerful tool for getting your needs met even when you are unable to self-direct care. These forms are generally free-of-charge and simple to complete without legal assistance. Contact your State Division of Health for information. Give a copy of the completed form to your primary physician, to principal family members and to each of your attorneys-in-fact. Keep the original at home with your "Emergency Medical Information" packet.

♦ **Keep documents handy.** Compile your medical documents including your Emergency Medical Information (which should include a complete list of your medications as well as emergency contacts) and your Living Will or Durable Power of Attorney for Health Care form. Put these in a large plastic bag and place it in a readily-accessible place such as taped to the inside of a cupboard door with a sign on the outside of the door saying "Emergency Medical Information Inside." The set of documents can be quickly grabbed in an emergency. Make sure all of your workers know this is here!

Emergency Help and Resources —

Call local hospitals to see what is available in your area. If none offer the service, national programs exist but usually at a higher cost. Most require a hook-up fee as well as monthly charges. Some funding sources underwrite the cost for participants. Check with local agencies or with your case worker, if you have one.

Few of us have (or want) round-the-clock PCAS watching over us. At the same time, we may risk injury or even death if left alone. Staying safe while alone is increased with the following solutions.

♦ **An emergency response unit** is a small alert system worn around your neck on a strap.

When needed, press the button and a dispatch center is notified. With a call box in your home, the dispatcher can talk to you and determine the degree of assistance needed. Designated friends, neighbors or family members are called to assist unless emergency personnel is needed.

Call local hospitals to see what is available in your area. If none offer the service, national programs exist but usually at a higher cost. Most require a hook-up fee as well as monthly charges. Some funding sources underwrite the cost for participants. Check with local agencies or with your case worker, if you have one.

Rare Pairs

♦ **A cordless or cell phone** kept nearby (such as in your wheelchair) is a vital solution to on-call help for many. If possible, program in important contacts. Most cell phone services offer free "911" calls.

♦ **Spare keys to your home or apartment** should be left with trusted family, friends, neighbors and/or PCAS in the event of an emergency. We're not surrendering our privacy by doing this, we're increasing our independence and safety. There's nothing quite as helpless as someone being at the door unable to get in if we call for help.

When hiding a spare key outside your house or apartment, don't put it under the door mat. One suggestion for apartment tenants is to discreetly tape a key above the door frame of a neighbor's door — but only with their permission. Let a couple people know where it is. This has been invaluable for me when new PCAS put me in the bathtub and leave the apartment to do the laundry, inadvertently locking the door behind them.

♦ **Home dwellers should leave their spare key** under a heavy object at a neighbor's house — not yours! Again, make sure it is a trusted neighbor and they gave permission to do this.

Hospitalization —

Don't think hospitalization can't happen to you. It has a nasty way of sneaking up on us all. Prepare now for the inevitable.

♦ **Don't wait too long to seek medical help** if you are sick or injured. Waiting will only make the situation worse.

♦ **Keep critical necessities handy** — including medications (prescription and over-the-counter), adaptive devices, special cushions, sponges, straws, and so forth. Make a list of essential items you would need in a hospital so they can be quickly gathered by a worker if needed.

- **Make a list of phone numbers** (and e-mail addresses) you may need in the hospital. Include common numbers (close family and friends) as well as PCAS, neighbors, landlord/manager, medical supply company, etc. Keep this with your medical documents. When I was in the hospital, the one number I needed most, but didn't have, was my live-in attendant's phone in her bedroom! I never had any reason to call her when I was home, but it was the only way to reach her when I was in the hospital.

- **Call ambulance companies** ahead of time to determine which would best meet your needs. Not all ambulances, for example, have electrical outlets in the vehicles for plugging in personal ventilators. Post that number by the phone for your PCA to quickly access.

- **ADA requires hospitals make essential services accessible.** Just as they must provide an interpreter for someone who is deaf, they must also do such things as modify the nurse call button if you can't press it. They must also absorb all costs for these services.

- **Ask which of your PCAS could assist you in the hospital.** Most of us need to provide much of our own help in the hospital due to special needs and short staff.

By being prepared for possible medical emergencies, you won't be caught in an ER drama of your own!

Chapter 18

Good Care Gone Bad

I always considered myself an excellent judge of character, a trait which has helped me to avoid hiring many "attendants from Hell." Such insights are not foolproof, however. Intentional deception or hidden neurosis can sometimes lead to getting more (or should I say less) than we bargained for.

Not long ago, I hired a woman who knocked my socks off with her warmth and friendliness. She equally impressed others including a close friend, also disabled, who was a professional counselor.

The worker seemed too good to be true. And, in fact, she was. In the end, I fired "Psycho Sally" but not without great deliberation and more than a little guilt. After all, she did pull me out of a jam by taking the job when she did, and she provided good care — in the beginning. But her Jeckyll-and-Hyde personality became increasingly evident and my care suffered severely for it. In retrospect, I should have fired her long before I did. But hindsight is always 20/20.

Although there were many justifications for firing someone, the line is seldom clear cut. Is tossing you in bed too hard "physical abuse"? Do you fire a PCA for "forgetting" to return the change after buying groceries? Is being two hours late grounds for dismissal? No doubt, we'd let these things slide. But what if they happen a second time? Or a third? When is enough enough? And at what point are we enabling them in their mistreatment of us?

> Gina ranted and raved because her live-in had been on a drunken binge for three weeks, leaving her without care. She complained that she had no money to pay for interim help. I asked what the problem was as she could simply take the funds she would have paid that live-in to hire someone else. "I can't do that!" she said, "I have to pay her for these weeks or she'll quit! Then where will I be?" The live-in returned and was paid. Shortly thereafter, she quit. When good care goes bad, we are often so enmeshed in the situation, we can't think clearly. After all, it's hard to keep our perspective when our safety net of care is shredding before our very eyes. We may have no emergency back-up or realize it takes weeks — or even months — to find a replacement. We're so desperate, we put up with anything because anything is better than nothing.

It's not unlike the battered wife who forgives the first slap, accepts an apology and believes it won't happen again. The situation worsens, but she feels it's easier to put up with a black eye and bruises than to make it on her own with three kids. Only when things become unbearable, does she take action.

We must not wait that long to take our own action. It is imperative we not let fear of abuse or abandonment supersede our better judgment. Remember, there was someone before this worker, and there will be someone after.

At the first sign of a problem, talk with the worker:

#1. Approach the problem with a clear head. Give yourself time for any anger to dissipate. Yelling will get you nowhere. You must remain calm for productive discussions to take place.

#2. Have back-up help ready before confronting the worker if you fear they may quit on the spot. This will give you the confidence to speak honestly.

#3. Choosing a right time and place is critical when discussing work issues. The setting must be:

- private
- quiet
- face-to-face

Turn off the TV and stereo and ask them to sit down so they are at your level. Remember, you are the employer. Don't, for example, expect to be viewed with authority while sitting on the commode! Discussions should take place when the PCA is not working and you are on equal grounds.

#4. Plan ahead. Spend time getting your thoughts together. What will you say? How might they respond? What will you say to their response? You may want to role play discussions with a friend.

#5. Begin with the positive before criticizing. "Chris, I really appreciate how well you clean my house. Unfortunately, your many last-minute calls to cancel have caused problems for me. I don't want to lose you, but if you can't be more reliable, I'll need to find someone else."

By telling the worker that they are valued, they're often more receptive to suggestions for change.

#6. Remain calm. Shouting and swearing will only heighten the tension and lessen the resolve. Never raise your voice to or above their level.

#7. Stay on track. The old "Your-mother-wears-Army-boots" line teaches us to stick to the issue at hand and not to bring up unrelated topics. If you are reprimanding the worker who is always late, don't interject how you can't stand their friends or that they forgot to charge your power chair the night before.

#8. Are workable solutions possible? A schedule change, clarification of needs, or more time off may be all it takes to resolve a problem. Ask if there's something you can do to improve the situation.

One night, while Sharon was putting me to bed, she said, "I think you need to find someone else to work for you." Although stunned, I calmly said, "Okay, if that's what you want." It was very late, I was in bed and realized this was not the time to discuss such a serious issue. She got me up early and rushed off to school. I spent the day making flyers advertising my need for immediate help.

That night when she returned she asked if I wanted her to leave. "NO!" I reassured her, "Of course not!" She then told me her only problem was that she wanted to study late at night down the hall from our apartment where there was a large table. "That's it? That's why you wanted to leave?" She responded, "You said I had to be here at night. I can't study in my room because I fall asleep."

We worked out a remote buzzer system that allowed her to work down the hall while allowing me to signal her if needed.

#9. If all else fails, ask if they want to leave. People who are unable to say they "want out" will sometimes sabotage the relationship, forcing you to fire them. This way they make you the bad guy, not themselves.

Unfortunately, not all problems can be resolved. Sometimes, we have no other choice but to fire the worker.

The act of firing an employee should never be taken lightly. It is a serious move — one which will effect you both. Never fire a worker without just cause, never do so on the spur of the moment, and never use firing as a power play.

Firing a live-in can cause tremendous anxiety for the disabled employer. It also can be dangerous. For this reason, it must be done with careful planning. Once again, follow an orderly procedure:

#1. First and foremost, ensure your safety. You are about to anger someone who is stronger than you are. Ensuring your safety is paramount when you tell them they are out of a job and a place to live.

#2. Never give notice of firing. Unfortunately, the PCA must not have the slightest hint we will fire them as our safety lies in the balance. Remain calm until you are in your wheelchair or otherwise as independent as possible before broaching the topic.

#3. Have someone with you when you fire the worker, if desired. You may want someone with you for moral support, as a witness, or to protect you if you suspect a violent response. If you rent, your landlord may be willing to be present.

#4. INSIST THAT THE LIVE-IN MOVES OUT IMMEDIATELY. You cannot live with a fired employee! They must be made to leave before the evening of the day they are fired. If they refuse, call the police who will assist in their removal.

#5. Remain present while they move out to ensure they do not damage or steal your property.

#6. Have the locks changed IMMEDIATELY. Your landlord may be willing to re-key the locks for you; otherwise, call a locksmith. Yes, it's ex-

110

pensive, but it's also worth every penny for the peace of mind gained. Don't hesitate doing this at the same time the live-in is moving out.

It should go without saying, it's best to have a back-up system in place before firing your primary caregiver. If possible, seek a replacement worker ahead of time by using a CIL, friend or family as the phone contact for ads. If no replacement is available, contact emergency back-up or respite workers prior to firing the worker to see who could help out on a part-time basis until a permanent worker can be found.

In a perfect world, we should never have to contend with sub-standard care. Emergency shelters and personal assistance services should be available until we are back on our feet (or wheels).

But sadly, this is seldom the case. We must sometimes contend with a bad situation until we can get out of it.

That is the key: we must never tolerate abuse or neglect and should always work toward getting out of these situations. No one deserves this, let alone physically-vulnerable people who are paying for this help!

Most PCAS are wonderful, caring people. With careful planning, your next one will be just such a gem.

Chapter 19

Rare Pairs

Our dream is to find that perfect someone who will provide us with care and companionship for life. Yet, as we go through one caregiver after another, it seems this dream can never be realized — by anyone.

Sometimes, however, the dream does come true...

Over the years, I've met an amazing array of parings managing to not only stay together for years but sometimes for life.

- ♦ Grace met Ben, a newly-injured patient, at a rehab hospital where she was on staff. She offered to became his live-in so he could leave the facility. She received no pay for months while they awaited supportive home care funding. Years later, they remain together having developed a strong, caring bond. Only declining health will ever force their separation.

- ♦ At age 12, Sam went to live with Frank who raised him like a son. Twenty-five years later, the tables have turned, and Sam became the caregiver of the 85-year-old man. Their love for each other was clearly evident in this one-of-a-kind, life-long relationship until Frank passed away earlier this year.

♦ Juan lived-in with his first charge for years until the man died. He has vowed to stay with his current employer just as long. Juan takes his live-in commitments seriously!

Special live-in relationships of this magnitude either happen or they don't but can't be planned. It's wrong to ever seek more than personal care from anyone you hire. While some disabled individuals hope to find a best friend, a lover, or a social companion in an employee, such relationships can't be found in help wanted ads. True friendships will evolve — or not — over time.

Even the epitome of loving relationships — marriage — often cannot hold up to the promise of staying together "in sickness and in health." Living and working together, day in and day out, when one spouse has a severe disability can place insurmountable stress on each partner often leading to its destruction. Making the relationship work, even under ideal conditions, requires exceptional communication and mutual respect.

Still, with all these barriers, there remain a fortunate few who evolve into perfect pairings. This does not mean the relationship is flawless, just that it works.

I've personally been blessed to have had some of my own. Hiring college students as my live-in PCAS, I realize longevity is unlikely. Most of the young women who commit to living with me do so for a year or less before graduating. Although not a life-long living situation, some remain special friends — sometimes more like adopted daughters — often for life. More than one have returned to visit saying it feels like they've come back home. There is no greater gift than these special bonds, yet they can never be predicted or planned.

So, at the height of live-in turnover, you may be encouraged to know that sometimes the dream does come true!

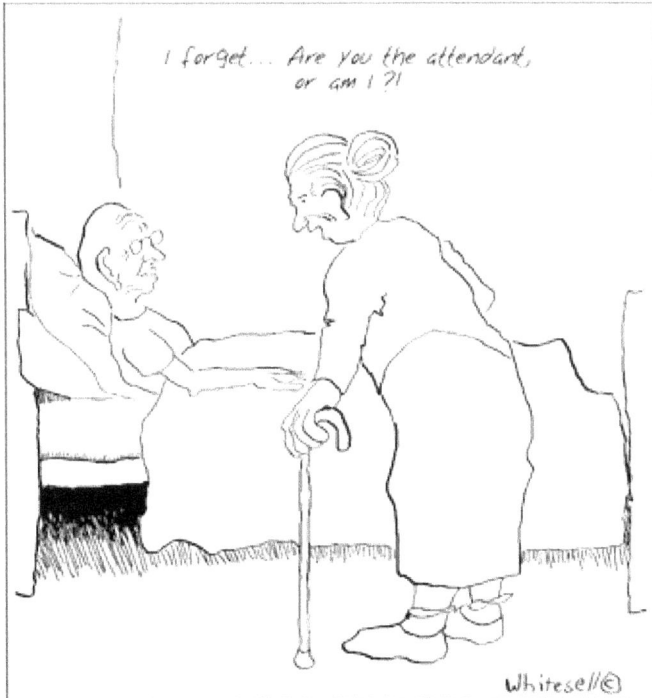

...not only stay together for years but sometimes for life.

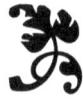

APPENDIX A

Sample Live-in Flier

Woman with Disability Seeks Live-in Attendant

FREE ROOM & $1300/mo.

Daytime hours free for school or work.

Furnished bedroom; quiet, security-locked apt. bldg.
(near Alverno College/Southgate/St. Luke's Hosp./Jackson Park)
Optional: Own phone line, cable TV in your room.

Your Prospective Roommate ➡

Active Woman with neuromuscular weakness.
Uses power chair; independent during the day.

Needs 45 min. personal care mornings & 1 hr. most nights.
—No cooking or heavy cleaning.—

"I love classic rock, animals, nature, my Mac computer."

No smoking allowed in apartment

PART-TIME
HELP ALSO SOUGHT
Occasional weekend nights;
Pays $70/night

IMMEDIATE OPENING!

You must be strong and able to fully
carry 95 lb. person for transfers.

For more details, interview and training,
call June at: ▮▮▮▮▮▮

Internet: PriceZRite@aol.com

I have a cat
named Cat

To live in with June. Call
To live in with June. Call
To live in with June. Call
To live in with June. Call
To live in with June. Call
To live in with June. Call
To live in with June. Call
To live in with June. Call
To live in with June. Call
To live in with June. Call
To live in with June. Call
To live in with June. Call
To live in with June. Call

APPENDIX B

Sample Newspaper Ad

LIVE-IN AIDE SOUGHT

by active disabled woman.

Room plus $1302/month. Days free. Ideal for students! Must be able to lift and carry 95 lbs.

Call ███████████ IMMEDIATELY

The three most common fee structures for newspaper ads are:

- ◆ per line
- ◆ per character (letters, numbers, punctuation, spaces);
- ◆ per word

Write your ad according to your local newspaper's fee structure to get the most for your money.

APPENDIX C

Sample Job Application

Job Application

Today's Date_____

Name_____

School Address_____

Permanent Address_____

Phone_____ Best time to call_____

Birthdate_____ Age_____

Soc. Sec. #_____

Valid driver's license_____

Name of college and major_____

Last three jobs, beginning with current:

Company	Phone	Supervisor	Dates worked
1._____	_____	_____	_____

Reason for leaving_____

| 2._____ | _____ | _____ | _____ |

Reason for leaving_____

| 3._____ | _____ | _____ | _____ |

Reason for leaving_____

List three personal references (no relatives or best friends):

Name   Phone   How you know them

1._____ _____ _____

2._____ _____ _____

3._____ _____ _____

Why do you want this job?_____

_____

_____

_____

Appendix D

Sample Live-in Contract

Live-In Attendant "Contract in Good Faith":

Rights & Responsibilities

We are about to enter into a unique working and living arrangement. The intent of this contract is to clarify the rights, responsibilities and expectations of this arrangement.

MY CARE

You are responsible for getting me up, dressed and out of bed each morning at a mutually agreed upon time. You also need to fix my breakfast drink as well as other short tasks as needed. Total time: approx. 30-45 min. You do not need to return until 9:00 p.m. unless otherwise agreed upon for non-bath nights. Night routines involve getting me ready for bed, commode use, and so forth; total time: approx. one hour.

On bath nights, you need to be here by 7:00 p.m. Bath, hair wash, brace care and laundry takes approx. 3 hours with time in between for your studies, etc.

You are also responsible for being on call during the night to turn me once/night, approx. 4 a.m. and for emergencies.

If you are going to be late any night, please call me. Just ask if you want or need to be late.

OTHER DUTIES

You are responsible for informing me when supplies and food are running low and need to be purchased (i.e. my orange juice, eggs, paper products, laundry detergent, laundry quarters.) You are not responsible for getting the items from the store; just inform me when they are needed.

CAT/FISH CARE

You are responsible for scooping the poop from the cat's litter box into the toilet as soon as you notice her smelly offering. You are not responsible for changing the litter box.

Discipline my cat only with a spray bottle of water or verbal commands. Physical abuse of my cat will not be tolerated.

The fish must be fed every other day along with turning the light on in the morning and off at night.

YOUR EMPLOYER

You are privately hired by me with funding by the Dept. of Health and Human Services with paychecks distributed from the accounting firm of ▇▇▇▇▇▇. **Your employer, for tax or other purposes, is "June Price."**

YOUR PAY

I am allocated $1302.00 per month for my care. Time sheets reflect 217 hours per month at $6.00/hour although this does not necessarily represent the actual time/hours you will work. Pay checks are scheduled to arrive on the 11th and 26th of each month. This is based on timely submission of time sheets (on the 15th and last day of each month). It is both of our responsibility to re-member to complete, sign and mail time sheets. We are both responsible for ensuring the accuracy of the times listed. If not done properly or timely, checks will be de-layed or rejected. I am not responsible if checks are de-layed by the County.

You may not get paid for days I am in a hospital.

You will not get paid when I am away to camp, unless you come as my caregiver.

You will not get paid when someone else is hired to work in your place.

There are no paid vacations, paid medical leave, etc. for you.

You have a right to unemployment compensation.

TIME OFF

You have the right to time off. We must work together to determine those days/dates/times. We can work to-gether to find another person to work in your place when you want time off, however the final decision as to who will work is mine. If a respite worker cannot be found, you will need to reschedule for another date. Advance requests of dates helps ensure back-up workers.

PERSONAL PROPERTY

I assume full responsibility for any damage I personally do to your property through accident or negligence. I will not assume responsibility for any damage to your prop-erty done by my cat. A closed bedroom door will prohibit her from entering if you choose for her to stay out. (She rarely causes damage of any kind.)

You have a right to put a key-operated lock on your bedroom door; however, management must be given a copy of the key.

I will respect your room and property and expect the same from you of mine.

YOUR ROOM

Your room must be kept pest and odor free. If you find insects in your room, you must report them to me immediately.

You must inform me of needed repairs in your room or if you have special needs, such as shelves or hooks.

You may paint your bedroom with management approval, a cash deposit to me, and other requirements. Ask if interested.

You may decorate you room as you wish within reason, however ask before mounting heavy items.

Use only new, heavy duty extension cords or electrical power strips if these are needed.

Burn candles safely, if at all; never leave unattended. You are responsible for any property damage resulting from your negligence.

Management will make a annual inspection of this apartment unit including your room for structural damage, repair needs and insect infestation. Neatness is irrelevant. You will receive prior notice of this.

Management has a right to enter this apartment, inc. your room, if illegal activities or health violations are suspected.

You have a right not to have respite workers sleep in your room or enter it at all.

When you move out, you are responsible for thoroughly cleaning your room (vacuuming, dusting, etc.).

134

YOUR MAIL

Your mail may be delivered to my mailbox. I will place your mail on "your" counter by the stove.

TELEPHONE

A separate phone line is installed in your room. You need to arrange for your own phone service.

CABLE T.V.

Cable TV is available in your room. You must pay for the hook-up and pay me $10/month for use **IF you want cable**.

KITCHEN PROCEDURES

You may use my microwave, can opener and other appliances in moderation. However, you are responsible for any damage or repair to these appliances resulting from your use or misuse.

Please provide your own dishes, glasses, cups, cooking utensils for the stove-top, oven and microwave as I have little. You may use my flatware as long as you do not take it out of the apartment (to school, etc.).

You are responsible for oven clean-up (including purchase of cleaning supplies) during your stay here and upon moving.

Please clean up your kitchen mess from cooking within a couple hours of use.

Please clean and put away any and all dishes by the end of each day; or place them out of my view.

All grains, flour, sugar and so forth must be kept in sealed, glass jars — no bags or boxes — to avoid insect infestation. Eat in your room if you wish, but don't leave food or food remains in there afterward. I have never had insect problems and don't want to start now.

GARBAGE

All food waste should be put down the garbage disposal whenever possible. When food cans or containers are empty, please rinse and recycle.

Stringy fruits and vegetables such as bananas and celery should be not be put down the disposal. Meat bones must be put in a plastic bag and taken outside to the trash to avoid smells and so my cat does not get at them. Trash is to be tied securely and taken out to the large dumpsters in the parking lot when you do this.

RECYCLE

Recycling is the law. Please put **rinsed** aluminum cans, glass bottles and #1 and #2 plastic in the designated paper bag in the kitchen; all paper products in the other. Break down cardboard boxes. There are also recycling containers outside by the dumpster.

BATHROOM — WET THINGS

Wet towels, clothing, wash clothes and rags should be hung flat to dry (not wadded up or thrown in a heap) to avoid mildew and odor.

UNIVERSAL PRECAUTIONS

Vinyl gloves are available for use for any personal care procedure you perform. Surgical masks are also available if you are sick. You have a right to use them for any and all procedures.

I PROVIDE/YOU PROVIDE

I will provide paper towels and toilet paper for normal use. You provide your own Kleenex and other paper products for other use (i.e. paper towels used to clean your car; etc.).

You provide all other supplies for personal use, including: light bulbs for your room, office/school supplies (Scotch tape, pens, etc.), kitchen supplies (plastic wrap, condiments, etc.) and so forth. You are welcome to use my cleaning products and vacuum to clean your room whenever you wish. Please make sure the vacuum does not pick up "junk" that may damage the unit. You will pay for repairs if you damage the vacuum.

You are expected to turn off all lights, fan, TV, etc., in your room before leaving for extended hours. Windows should be kept open no more than a crack on cold days to avoid excessive heating bills.

You will be charged for damage or breakage anything of mine or the apartment's property that you do out of negligence.

VAN USE

If we both feel comfortable, you can drive me in my van. You are never to use my van without my permission.

OVERNIGHT GUESTS

Occasional overnight guests are welcome as long as you clear it with me beforehand. They may use the sofa sleeper or stay in your room. Male guests may stay overnight in your room as long as discretion is employed and respect for each of our privacy is given. Children may visit if they are quiet and nondestructive.

SMOKING

Smoking by you or your guests is strictly prohibited in this apartment at any and all times, even when I am not here. Smoking is also prohibited in the common areas of the apartment building (hallways, elevator, stairwell). Smoking **is allowed** in apartments of consenting tenants as well as outside. Proper outside disposal of butts is appreciated.

ALCOHOL

Moderate, responsible consumption of alcohol in this apartment by you and/or your guests is acceptable if you are over 21.

No one is allowed in this apartment while intoxicated or high.

You must be straight and sober when working for me, including during the night when I might call.

ILLICIT DRUGS

Possession or use of illicit drugs by you or your guests in this apartment is strictly prohibited and may be grounds for immediate dismissal.

POLICE RECORD

I may run a police check on you and reserve the right to fire or not hire you based on the results.

GROUNDS FOR IMMEDIATE DISMISSAL:

- Gross negligence of job responsibilities.
- Police record which I deem unacceptable.
- Possession or use of illicit drugs on this property by you or your guests.
- Working while intoxicated or high.
- Theft of any type or degree.
- Unauthorized use of my van.

- Physical or verbal abuse toward myself or my cat.
- Unreported pregnancy.
- Blatant lies and deception.
- Actions which result in warnings from management.

NON-RIGHTS

You do not have a right to have another person or people permanently staying with you here in this apartment.

You do not have the right to own or keep a pet here.

You do not have a right to disseminate copies of your apartment keys.

State law does **not** require that I give you any notice before firing you. As my live-in attendant, free rent is a "perk" which goes with this job and therefore I am under no legal obligation to give you a 30-day notice to find other housing if fired.

RESIGNATION

If you choose to leave, please keep in mind that it has taken me an average of two months to find a replacement attendant. Please be respectful of my dilemma and allow me as much lead time as possible to locate, train and hire your replacement.

FORWARDING OF MAIL AND TAX FORMS

The responsibility for putting in a forwarding address with the post office is YOURS. After you leave, I will return to sender any first-class mail that comes here if no forwarding address is on file. Non-first class mail will be discarded.

Your tax forms will be mailed to me by January 31 of next year. If I have no forwarding address for you, you are responsible for picking up the forms before April 15. After that date, I will return them to the accounting firm.

MANAGEMENT RULES

According to my lease, I am totally responsible for your actions.

Smoking is not allowed in the common areas of this building.

All garbage must be tightly secured in plastic bags and placed in the outside trash bin. Do not overflow garbage cans.

Auto repairs and car washing are not allowed in the parking lot.

Lot parking is allowed on a first-come, first-serve basis in Visitor spots only. When full, you or your guests must seek street parking. Illegally parked vehicles will be towed at owner's expense.

You are not allowed to prop open an outside locked, security door.

ABOVE AND BEYOND...

Above and beyond all of the aforementioned, it is imperative we show each other respect, courtesy, dignity and honesty. Without these, none of the above matters.

I fully understand this "contract in good faith" and will adhere it.

Live-in's Name_____ Date_____

June Price_____ Date_____

TIPS, & THINGS YOU'LL NEED

Your mailing address will be

██████████████████████████.

The apartment number is critical to ensure your getting mail.

When friends come to visit, let them know your name does NOT appear on the tenant listing. They should be told to locate "Price" and ring this apartment number.

For your room, you may want to bring:

♦ a TV.

♦ table and/or floor lamp(s)

♦ a fan for Summer

Halogen lamps are **prohibited** as they are a known fire hazard.

You may re-organize your bedroom furniture and may prefer to do so before you move everything in. Furniture placement is somewhat limited.

If you have a bike, you can keep it locked outside in the designated area or left in your room but not in the living room.

Ask me to show you where the emergency pull cord is in your room. It's taped up so no one will accidentally pull it.

The heat in your room is "off," but you may turn it as high as needed.

Washers require 75¢ each load and run 25 min. Dryers require 75$ and run 1 hour. You may use the upstairs or downstairs laundry room. The laundry room opens at 8:00 a.m. and locks at 11:00 p.m. daily.

I have heavy, white drapes for your bedroom window. Let me know if you want them. If you want other window coverings, clear it with me beforehand as there are lease restrictions regarding this.

If you accidentally lock yourself out of this apartment, Sandy in #102 has a key.

APPENDIX E

Emergency Medical Information

Emergency Medical Information

Personal information: [name, address]

Phone:

Birthdate:

Height:

Weight:

Social Security Number:

Medical Insurance:

Primary Disability:

Secondary Disability:

Drug Allergies:

Other Allergies:

Prescription Medications:

Over-the-counter Drugs:

Dietary Restrictions:

Recent hospitalization/illnesses:

Primary Physician:

[Additional physicians]:

Durable Power of Attorney for Health Care:

Emergency Contacts:

This Information was last updated on:

APPENDIX F

Resources

Magazines for People with Disabilities

When I was about ten years old, an older, disabled neighbor rolled his wheelchair to my parents' home and handed me a copy of ACCENT On Living magazine. It was the first disability-oriented publication I ever read. Without question, it opened my world to an awareness that there were more than disabled children in the world (as special schools and telethons had led me to believe) and that many of us would grow up to be disabled adults who had the potential of being employed, married or college-educated. We had, after all, no role models back then, no images of what we could become. ACCENT — and all the publications which followed — provided proof that we could have a future — and a bright one at that!

Publications geared to the disabled community are invaluable in providing information, networking and support to others with similar abilities and needs. If you have not already done so, you may wish to examine some of the more notable magazines currently published in the United States which focus on the lives and needs of individuals who have physical disabilities.

Magazine descriptions are those of the individual publications'. Subscriptions are for 12 issues per year unless otherwise stated. Rates are for one year though most offer discounts for two- or three-year commitments. The currency requested for foreign subscriptions is US dollars. Some publications offer a free sample issue to readers upon request.

ACCENT On Living

Magazine and service for, by and about people who happen to have a disability. Serving the physically disabled community since 1956.
Published quarterly
$12 - US
$16 - Int'l, inc. Canada and Mexico
ACCENT on Living
P.O. Box 700
Bloomington, IL 61702-0700
Phone:
800/787-8444
309/378-2961
Internet: http://www.blvd.com/accent/
E-mail: acntlvng@aol.com

Enable Magazine

Features articles and chat that target the interests of active people with disabilities and explores ideas and opportunities for making life more enjoyable for people with disabilities and their families.
The $19.95 price of the bimonthly publication also enrolls you as a member of the American Association of People with Disabilities.
Enable Magazine
3659 Cortea Road, Suite 110
Bradenton, FL 34210
Phone: 888/4-ENABLE (888/436-2253)
Internet: http://www.enable-magazine.com/enable_online_magazine_grafic.htm
E-mail: readenable@aol.com

New Mobility

New Mobility is the monthly disability culture, resources and lifestyle magazine for, by and of people with disabilities. Look for an irreverent style and an insider point of view that takes no prisoners.

$27.95 – US $35.95 - Canada
$57.95 - Int'l (surface) $117.95 - Int'l (air-mail)
New Mobility
P.O. Box 491861
Los Angeles, CA 90049
Phone: 888/850-0344
Internet: http://www.newmobility.com/
E-mail: marilyn@miramar.com
 contact New Mobility at:
No Limits Communications, Inc.
PO Box 220
Horsham, PA 19044
Phone: 800/675-9134

Paraplegia News

The news and information magazine for people with mobility impairments covering the latest on spinal cord injury research, new products, legislation, people with disabilities, accessible travel, computers, and more.

$23 - US $32 - International
PN/Paraplegia News
2111 E. Highland Ave, Suite 180
Phoenix, AZ 85016
Phone: (888) 888-2201
Phone: 888/888-2201
or (602) 224-0500 for int'l callers
Internet: http://www.pva.org/index.htm

E-mail: pvapub@aol.com

Ragged Edge

Ragged Edge is the successor to the award-winning periodical, The Disability Rag. In Ragged Edge you'll find the best in today's writing about society's "ragged edge" issues: medical rationing, genetic discrimination, assisted suicide, long-term care, attendant services. We cover the disability experience in America — what it means to be a crip living at the end of the 20th century.
$17.50 - US
$35 - for institutions
$42 - Int'l including Canada and Mexico
Ragged Edge
P.O. Box 145
Louisville, KY 40201
Phone: 502/894-9492
Internet: http://www.ragged-edge-mag.com/index.shtml#edge
E-mail: editor@ragged-edge-mag.com or Edge-Mag@aol.com
Sports 'n Spokes: The magazine of wheelchair sports and recreation for the active wheeler.
Published 8 times/year
$21 - US
$27 - International

Sports 'n Spokes

2111 E. Highland Ave, Suite 180
Phoenix, AZ 85016
Phone: 888-888-2201
or (602) 224-0500 for int'l callers
Internet: http://www.pva.org/sns/index.htm
E-mail: snsmagaz@aol.com

ABOUT THE NATIONAL COUNCIL ON INDEPENDENT LIVING

Founded in 1982, the National Council on Independent Living (NCIL) is the national membership association of centers for independent living (CILs) and people with disabilities. NCIL, as the only national, cross-disability, grassroots organization run by and for people with disabilities, has been instrumental in efforts to standardize requirements for consumer control in advocacy, management and delivery of services provided through CILs.

Until 1992, NCIL's efforts to foster consumer control and direction in independent living services were coordinated through an extensive network of volunteers from CILs and other organizations around the country. Since 1992, NCIL has had a national office in Arlington, Virginia, just minutes from Washington, D.C.. While NCIL continues to rely on the commitment and dedication of volunteers from around the country, the establishment of a national office has strengthened its capacity for eliminating discrimination and unequal treatment based on disability. Today, NCIL is a strong voice for independent living in our nation's capital.

With your participation, NCIL can continue delivering the message of independent living to those individuals who are charged with the responsibility of making laws and creating programs designed to assure equal rights for all.

153

NCIL'S MISSION:
 NCIL promotes a national advocacy agenda that advances:
1. the full integration and equal participation of people with disabilities in society, and
2. the development, improvement and expansion of centers for independent living.

NCIL Central Office Resources
1916 Wilson Blvd., Suite 209
Arlington, VA 22201
703/525-3406 (V)
703/5254153 (TTY)
703/525-3409 (FAX)
ncil@tsbbs08 .tnet.com (E-mail)
Laural Richards
Independent Living Research Utilization (ILRU)
2323 South Shepard, Suite #1000
Houston, TX 77019
Research & Training Center on Rural Rehabilitation
The University of Montana
52 Corbin Flail
Missoula, MT 59812

NCIL Regional Representatives

CHAIR: Jan Day
Center for Accessible Living, Inc.
981 S. Third Street, Suite 102
Louisville, KY 40203-2261
502/589-6620 (V)   502/589-3980 (TTY)

502/589-3980 (FAX)   janday (DIMENET)
janday@callou.winnet (E-mail)

REGION 1
Larry Robinson   (No Alternate)
Granite State IL Foundation
172 Pembroke Road
P.O. Box 7268
Concord, NH 03301-7268
603/228-9680 (V)
603/228-9680 (TTY)
603/225-3304 (FAX)
gsilf (DIMENET)

REGION 2
June Roberts (No Alternate)
Self Initiated Living Options, Inc.
745 Waverly Avenue
Holtsville, NY 11742
516/654-8007 (Y)
516/654-8076 (TTY)
516/654-8077 (FAX)

REGION 3	REGION 3 ALTERNATE
Kathleen Kleinmann	Frank Pinter
Tn-County Partnership for IL Inc.	Maryland CIL,
69 E. Beau Street Road	5807 Hartford
Washington, PA 15301 21214	Baltimore, MD
412/223-5115 (V)	410/444-1400 (V)

155

412/223-5115 (TTY)   800/735-2258
(TTY)
412/223-5119 (FAX)   410/444-0825
(FAX)
kleinman (DIMENET)   mcil (DIMENET)

REGION 4
Jan Day   (No Alternate)
Center for Accessible Living, Inc.
981 S. Third Street. Suite 102
Louisville, KY 40203-2261
502/589-6620 (V)
502/589-3980 (TTY)
502/589-3980 (FAX)
janday (DIMENET)
janday@callou.win.net (E-mail)

REGION 5
Steven K. Thovson   (No Alternate)
Southwestern CIL
109 S. Fifth Street, Suite 700
Marshall, MN 56258
507/532-2221 (V)
507/532-2221 (TTY)
507/532-2222 (FAX)
SWCIL@polaristel.net (E-mail)

REGION 6
Carri George (No Alternate)
ILRU
2323 S. Shepherd, Suite 1000
Houston, TX 77019

713/520-0232 (V)
713/520-5785 (TTY)
713/520-5136 (FAX)
cgeorge (DIMENET)

REGION 7
Michael Oxford
Topeka ILRC
Rights
501 SW Jackson, Suite 100
Topeka, KS 66603
Street
913/233-4572 (V)
52245
913/233-4572 (TTY)
913/233-1561 (FAX)
(TTY)
mlox (DIMENET)
(FAX)

REGION 7 ALTERNATE
Casey Hayes
Evert Conner

& Resources CIL
20 East Market

Iowa City, IA

319/338-3870 (V)
319/338-3870

319/338-8385

REGION 8
Nancy Conklin
Center for Independence

1600 Ute Avenue, Suite 100
St
Grand Junction, CO 81501

970/241-7330 (V)

REGION 8 ALTERNATE
Debra Mair
Utah Independent
Living Center, Inc.
3445 South Main

Salt Lake City, UT
84115
801/466-5565 (V)

970/241-8130 (TTY)   801/466-9910
(TTY)
970/245-3341 (FAX)   801/466-2363
(FAX)
nconklinl @juno.com
        uilc@xmission.com

REGION 9
Kent Mickelson   (No Alternate)
Center for Independence of the Disabled
875 O'Neill Avenue
Belmont, CA 94002-3837
650/595-0783 (V)
650/595-0743 (TTY)
650/595-0261 (FAX)

REGION 10
Kelly Buckland   (No Alternate)
Idaho SILC
P. 0. Box 83720
350 N. 9th Street, Suite 610-B
Boise, ID 83720-9601
208/334-3800 (V)
208/334-3800 (TTY)
208/334-3 803 (FAX)
idasilc (DIMENET)
kbucklan@silc.state.id.us

About the Illustrator

Barry Whitesell is a graphic artist living near Poughkeepsie, NY. Formally trained as a fine artist at the State University of New York at Albany, he has worked as an illustrator, cartoonist, and graphic/web designer. Born in 1963, he said he spends much of his free time trying to decide if he is a "Baby-Boomer" or a "Generation X'er."

Barry is intimately familiar with the trials and tribulations of hiring and working with PCAs. As a result of having spinal muscular atrophy, he uses a power chair full-time and requires assistance with most aspects of daily living. Having known both "attendants from Hell" and "attendants from Heaven," the concept for the cover illustration came naturally to him. Currently, Barry is working on supplementing his mother's excellent full-time assistance an arrangement consisting of room and board in exchange for care.

Barry is always accepting commissions for new design and illustration projects, as well as applications for the live-in position. He can be reached by e-mail at: Barry@WhitesellEnterprises.com, or by phone at 914.227.6593.

About the Author

June Price was born in 1947 with spinal muscular atrophy, type II (SMA-II), a rare, neuromuscular disease. Never able to walk, she relies on a power chair and needs assistance with all her personal care. June lived with her parents until February, 1980, at which time she became one of the first physically disabled adults in Milwaukee, Wisconsin, to move into a wheelchair accessible, low-income apartment complex for disabled and elderly people.

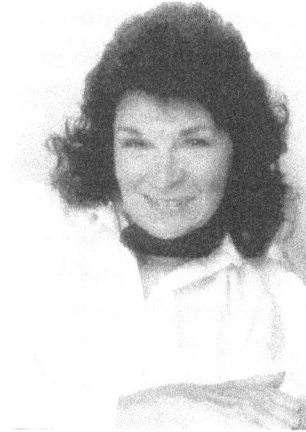

Initially, June only needed PCAs to come in for her care morning and night, as she was able to manage on her own during the day (albeit with tremendous effort). These workers were neighborhood woman with small children who welcomed cash payments and short work hours. She met toileting needs with an external, urinary device she co-invented and still uses today.

In 1988, June moved into a new apartment complex geared to people with physical disabilities. A two-bedroom apartment made it possible to hire a live-in attendant as she now needed nighttime repositioning. College students were a perfect fit for this position which offered housing, salary and days free for outside work or school.

By 1995, home health aides were brought into the equation for mealtime and toileting assistance. Unlike the privately-hired overnight workers, the home health aides are agency-hired, and the case is managed by a nurse.

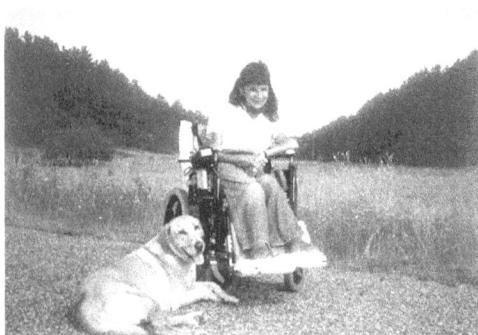

Since 1991, June has used a BiPAP S/T ventilator with a nasal mask to help her breathe during the night. In 2000, she had a PLV-100 volume ventilator put on her wheelchair which she uses as needed with a mouthpiece attachment.

As her care needs have increased, she reduces the potential of worker burnout by hiring three college students to share the weekly, overnight schedule, each working 1-3 nights per week, in lieu of one live-in. (See Chapter 14 for "The 'Live-Out' Live-In."

June's literary credits include articles for New Mobility and MDA's Quest. She founded and edited Living SMArt, an international newsletter for people with spinal muscular atrophy.

www.ingramcontent.com/pod-product-compliance
Lightning Source LLC
Chambersburg PA
CBHW050120210326
41519CB00015BA/4042